Fluids & Electrolytes

JUST THE FACTS

Fluids & Electrolytes

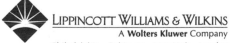
LIPPINCOTT WILLIAMS & WILKINS
A **Wolters Kluwer** Company

Philadelphia • Baltimore • New York • London
Buenos Aires • Hong Kong • Sydney • Tokyo

STAFF

Executive Publisher
Judith A. Schilling McCann, RN, MSN

Editorial Director
William J. Kelly

Clinical Director
Joan M. Robinson, RN, MSN

Senior Art Director
Arlene Putterman

Editorial Project Manager
Elizabeth P. Lowe

Clinical Project Manager
Beverly Ann Tscheschlog, RN, BS

Editor
Nancy Priff

Clinical Editor
Tamara M. Kear, RN, MSN, CNN

Copy Editors
Kimberly Bilotta (supervisor),
Lisa Stockslager, Kelly Taylor

Designers
Debra Moloshok (project manager),
Will Boehm (book design),
Jacalyn Facciolo (cover design)

Digital Composition Services
Diane Paluba (manager),
Joyce Rossi Biletz, Donna S. Morris

Manufacturing
Patricia K. Dorshaw (director),
Beth J. Welsh

Editorial Assistants
Megan Aldinger, Carol Caputo,
Tara Carter-Bell, Linda Ruhf

Indexer
Barbara Hodgson

JTFF&E - D N O S A J
06 05 04   10 9 8 7 6 5 4 3 2 1

Library of Congress
Cataloging-in-Publication Data
Just the facts : fluids & electrolytes.
    p. ; cm.
  Includes bibliographical references and index.
    ISBN 1-58255-340-8 (alk. paper)
    1. Water-electrolyte imbalances—Nursing—Handbooks, manuals, etc. 2. Water-electrolyte balance (Physiology)—Handbooks, manuals, etc. I. Lippincott Williams & Wilkins. II Title: Fluids & electrolytes.
    [DNLM: 1. Water-Electrolyte Imbalance—nursing—Handbooks. 2. Water-Electrolyte Balance—physiology—Handbooks. WD 220 J96 2005]
RC630.J87 2005
616.3'992—dc22   2004005311

Contents

Contributors and consultants

Jane Banton, RN, BSN, CRNI
I.V. Therapy Coordinator
University of Wisconsin
  Hospital and Clinics
Madison

Peggy Bozarth, RN, MSN
Professor
Hopkinsville (Ky.) Community
  College

Jeanette K. Chambers, RN, PhD
Program Manager, Nursing
  Research & Magnet
  Recognition
Riverside Methodist Hospital
Columbus, Ohio

Merry Jahn Chandler, RN, BSN,
  MA, MSN
Assistant Professor
McNeese State University
  College of Nursing
Lake Charles, La.

Arlene M. Coughlin, RN, MSN
Nursing Faculty
Holy Name Hospital School of
  Nursing
Teaneck, N.J.

Linda Evans, RN, BSN, CDE
Nurse Educator, Wound Care
Helen Keller Hospital
Sheffield, Ala.

Nancy H. Haynes, RN, MS, CCRN
Assistant Professor of Nursing
Saint Luke's College
Kansas City, Mo.

Peggy Jenkins, RN, BS, MS, CCRN
Associate Professor of Nursing
Hartwick College
Oneonta, N.Y.

JoAnne Konick-McMahan, RN,
  MSN, CCRN
Instructor, School of Nursing
Reading (Pa.) Hospital and
  Medical Center
Staff Nurse, MICU/Stepdown
Hospital of the University of
  Pennsylvania
Philadelphia

Nancy L. Kranzley, RN, MS
Pulmonary Clinical Nurse
  Specialist
Cincinnati Therapy Centers

Linda McGovern, RN, MSN, CNN, CCTC
Clinical Transplant Coordinator
Lehigh Valley Hospital
Allentown, Pa.

Catherine T. Milne, APRN, MSN, BC, CWOCN, NP-C
Advanced Practice Nurse
Connecticut Clinical Nursing
Associates, LLC
Bristol

Janet L. Parker, RN, CS, MSN, CCP, FNP
Assistant Chief, Perfusion
Deborah Heart and Lung Center
Brown Mills, N.J.

Marlene Roman, RN, ARNP, MSN, CMSRN
*Medical-Surgical Clinical Nurse
Specialist*
North Broward Medical Center
Pompano Beach, Fla.

Patricia Shatney, APRN, MSN, CNN
Nephrology Nurse Practitioner
Nephrology Associates
Bridgeport, Conn.

Concha Carrillo Sitter, CGRN, MS, APN, FNP
*Gastroenterology Nurse
Practitioner*
Sterling (Ill.) Rock Falls Clinic

Patricia D. Weiskittel, RN, MSN, CNN, CS, ARNP
*Renal Transplant Clinical Nurse
Specialist*
University Hospital
Cincinnati

Kate Willcutts, RD, MS, CNSD
*Clinical Instructor/Surgical
Nutrition Support Nutritionist*
University of Virginia
Charlottesville

Foreword

Throughout history, medicine has been dealing with homeostasis, from balancing the four humors—blood, yellow bile, phlegm, and black bile—to managing the complex fluid and electrolyte balance of acutely ill patients. Now that the demand on nurses is higher than ever and typical hospitalized patients are much sicker than in the past, a concise, easy-to-read, and easy-to-use reference book is essential. You'll find that *Just the Facts: Fluids & Electrolytes* is well organized, and the information is easy to synthesize. It's a valuable tool that can be used by both the seasoned and the novice nurse in any health care setting.

The best feature of this book is that it's succinct. Short bullet points immediately draw attention to signs and symptoms and to management—the critical information that a nurse needs right away. Other helpful features are the flowcharts explaining pathophysiology and highlighted text boxes listing drugs. The pathophysiology flowcharts outline the progression of the imbalance, ending with the signs and symptoms the patient will exhibit. Especially helpful are the bulleted lists of drugs that can affect the particular imbalance. When a specific piece of information is critical, it is flagged with an *Alert* logo. Information relevant to different age groups is indicated by an *Age alert* logo.

The first chapter, Balancing basics, discusses balancing fluids, electrolytes, and acids and bases in the body. Chapter 2, Fluid imbalances, outlines pathophysiology, causes, signs and symptoms, diagnostic test results, and management of dehydration, hypervolemia, and hypovolemia. Chapter 3, Electrolyte imbalances, covers high and low levels of each electrolyte, including a short definition of each level, the most severe symptoms that each imbalance will cause, pathophysiology, causes (including drugs that can cause the imbalance), signs and symptoms, and management of the imbalance. Chapter 4, Acid and base imbalances, covers respiratory acidosis and alkalosis and metabolic acidosis and alkalosis. Chapter 5, Disorders that cause imbalances, addresses heart failure, respiratory failure, excessive GI fluid loss, renal failure, syndrome of inappropriate antidiuretic hormone secretion, and burns. The last chapter, Treating imbalances, focuses on I.V. fluid replacement therapy, total parenteral nutrition, dialysis, and transfusions.

This book is the first in the *Just the Facts* series. The compact size of this book, the one-column format, the bulleted-list style, and the special alerts and age alerts make this a very effective reference. As a busy nurse, I need to know that there are references that are to the point, so that I can provide the best possible care to my patients. I know that the status of patients can change rapidly, and this tool will enable me to "balance" the situation. No matter what area of nursing you work in, patients with electrolyte imbalances will be a part of your practice, so be prepared.

Lynda K. Ball, RN, BS, BSN, CNN
Quality Improvement Coordinator
Northwest Renal Network
Seattle, Wash.

1

Balancing basics

Fluid balance

◆ Nearly all major organs in the body work together to maintain a balance of daily fluid gains and losses.

◆ Insensible fluid losses occur through the skin and lungs; they're called insensible because they can't be seen or measured.

◆ Sensible fluid losses occur through urination, defecation, and wounds; they're called sensible because they can be perceived and measured.

◆ The body holds intracellular fluid inside the cells (in the intracellular compartment) and outside the cells (in the extracellular compartment).

◆ To maintain balance, fluid distribution between the intracellular and extracellular compartments must remain constant.

◆ Extracellular fluid includes interstitial fluid, which surrounds the cells, and intravascular fluid (plasma), which is the liquid portion of blood.

◆ Fluid distribution varies with age. Infants store a greater percentage of body water in the interstitial spaces than adults do.

 AGE ALERT *The risk of fluid imbalance increases with age because muscle mass decreases and the proportion of fat increases over the years.*

Fluid types

◆ Body fluids may appear in isotonic, hypotonic, or hypertonic solutions.

◆ An isotonic solution has the same solute concentration as another solution.

◆ Fluid doesn't shift between isotonic solutions because they're equally concentrated and already in balance.

ISOTONIC SOLUTION

The solute concentration of an isotonic solution is about equal to that of serum. Therefore, it stays in the intravascular space after administration.

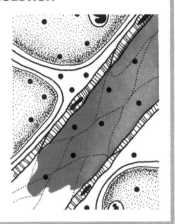

♦ A hypotonic solution has a lower solute concentration than another solution.
♦ When a less concentrated (hypotonic) solution is placed next to a more concentrated solution, fluid shifts from the hypotonic solution into the more concentrated compartment to equalize the concentrations.

HYPOTONIC SOLUTION

The solute concentration of a hypotonic solution is less than that of serum. Therefore, it shifts out of the intravascular compartment after administration.

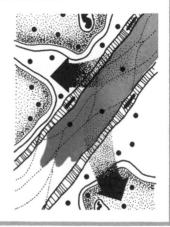

◆ A hypertonic solution has a higher solute concentration than another solution.

◆ Although a hypertonic solution has more solutes than an adjacent solution, it has less fluid.

◆ Fluid tends to move out of the less concentrated solution into the more concentrated (hypertonic) solution until both solutions have the same amount of solutes and fluid.

HYPERTONIC SOLUTION

The solute concentration of a hypertonic solution is higher than that of serum. Therefore, it draws fluid into the intravascular space after administration.

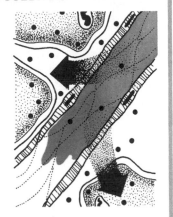

Fluid movement

◆ Fluids and solutes constantly move within the body to maintain homeostasis.
◆ Solutes move through intracellular, interstitial, and intravascular compartments by crossing semipermeable membranes.
◆ Movement occurs through cells and capillaries.

Movement through cells

◆ In diffusion, solutes move from an area of higher concentration to an area of lower concentration, which requires no energy.

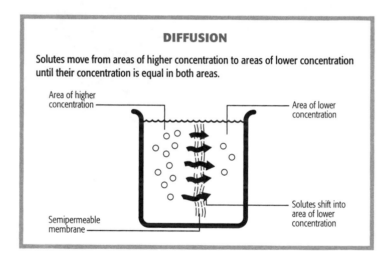

DIFFUSION

Solutes move from areas of higher concentration to areas of lower concentration until their concentration is equal in both areas.

Area of higher concentration

Area of lower concentration

Solutes shift into area of lower concentration

Semipermeable membrane

◆ In active transport, solutes move from an area of lower concentration to an area of higher concentration, which requires energy.

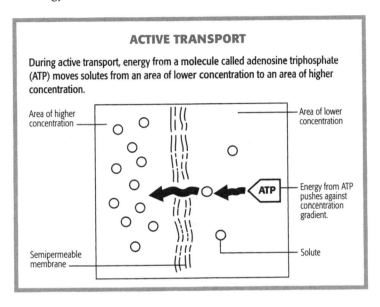

ACTIVE TRANSPORT

During active transport, energy from a molecule called adenosine triphosphate (ATP) moves solutes from an area of lower concentration to an area of higher concentration.

Area of higher concentration

Area of lower concentration

Energy from ATP pushes against concentration gradient.

ATP

Semipermeable membrane

Solute

◆ In osmosis, fluid moves passively from an area with more fluid and fewer solutes to an area with less fluid and more solutes.

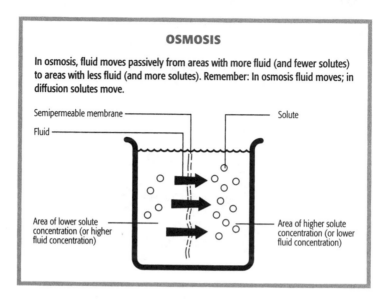

OSMOSIS

In osmosis, fluid moves passively from areas with more fluid (and fewer solutes) to areas with less fluid (and more solutes). Remember: In osmosis fluid moves; in diffusion solutes move.

Semipermeable membrane

Fluid

Solute

Area of lower solute concentration (or higher fluid concentration)

Area of higher solute concentration (or lower fluid concentration)

Movement through capillaries

- Capillaries have walls thin enough to let solutes pass through.
- Fluids and solutes move through capillary walls to help maintain fluid balance.
- Hydrostatic pressure (the pressure of blood pushing against capillary walls) forces fluids and solutes through the walls.

FLUID MOVEMENT THROUGH CAPILLARY WALLS

When hydrostatic (fluid-pushing) pressure builds inside a capillary, it forces fluids and solutes out through the capillary walls into the interstitial fluid.

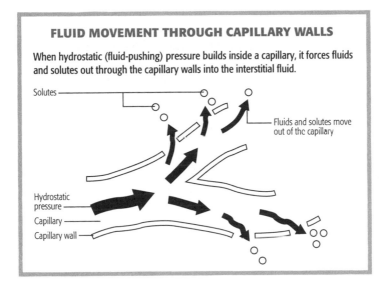

Solutes

Fluids and solutes move out of the capillary

Hydrostatic pressure

Capillary

Capillary wall

◆ When the hydrostatic pressure inside a capillary is greater than the pressure in the surrounding interstitial space, fluids and solutes inside the capillary are forced into the interstitial space.

◆ When the pressure inside a capillary is less than the pressure outside it, fluids and solutes move back into the capillary.

◆ Reabsorption prevents an excessive amount of fluid from leaving the capillaries.

◆ Within the capillaries, albumin acts like a water magnet to attract and hold water inside the vessel.

◆ The pulling force of albumin is known as the plasma colloid osmotic pressure.

◆ As long as hydrostatic pressure exceeds plasma colloid osmotic pressure, water and solutes can leave the capillaries and enter the interstitial fluid.

◆ When hydrostatic pressure falls below plasma colloid osmotic pressure, water and solutes return to the capillaries.

Maintaining fluid balance

◆ The kidneys and various hormones and mechanisms work together to maintain fluid balance.

◆ A problem in any of these things can cause a fluid imbalance.

Kidneys

◆ In the kidneys, nephrons filter about 180 L of blood daily; this amount is the glomerular filtration rate.

◆ Nephrons produce 1 to 2 L of urine daily.

◆ The kidneys conserve water or excrete excess fluid to maintain balance.

◆ The minimum excretion rate varies with age.

 AGE ALERT *Infants and young children excrete urine at a higher rate than adults because they have higher metabolic rates and because their kidneys are less efficient than adults' kidneys are until about age 2.*

Antidiuretic hormone

◆ Antidiuretic hormone (ADH), or vasopressin, regulates fluid balance.

◆ ADH restores blood volume by reducing diuresis and increasing water retention.

HOW ANTIDIURETIC HORMONE WORKS

Antidiuretic hormone (ADH) regulates fluid balance through a series of steps, which are outlined here.

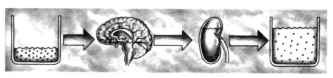

The hypothalamus senses low blood volume and increased serum osmolality and signals the pituitary gland.

The pituitary gland secretes ADH into the bloodstream.

ADH causes the kidneys to retain water.

Water retention boosts blood volume and decreases serum osmolality.

Renin-angiotensin-aldosterone system

◆ This mechanism helps maintain a balance of sodium and water and a healthy blood volume and pressure.

◆ When the fluid or sodium level falls, juxtaglomerular cells secrete renin, which stimulates angiotensin II production.

◆ Angiotensin II causes vasoconstriction and stimulates aldosterone production.

◆ Aldosterone causes sodium and water retention, leading to increased fluid volume and sodium levels.

◆ When the blood pressure returns to normal, the body halts the release of renin, which stops this system.

HOW ALDOSTERONE WORKS

Aldosterone, produced as a result of the renin-angiotensin mechanism, acts to regulate fluid volume as described below.

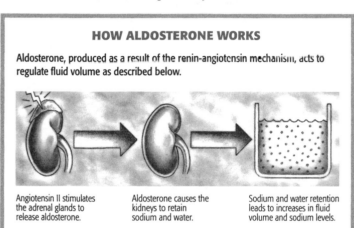

| Angiotensin II stimulates the adrenal glands to release aldosterone. | Aldosterone causes the kidneys to retain sodium and water. | Sodium and water retention leads to increases in fluid volume and sodium levels. |

Atrial natriuretic peptide

- Atrial natriuretic peptide (ANP) is a cardiac hormone.
- The actions of ANP oppose those of the renin-angiotensin-aldosterone system.
- ANP decreases blood pressure and reduces intravascular blood volume.
- Atrial stretching increases the amount of ANP released.

Thirst mechanism

- Thirst results from even small losses of fluid.
- When oral mucous membranes become dry, they stimulate the thirst center in the hypothalamus.

Electrolyte balance

- ◆ Electrolytes work with fluids to maintain health and well-being.
- ◆ Electrolytes are substances that, when in solution, separate into electrically charged particles called ions.
- ◆ Anions are electrolytes that produce a negative charge; cations are electrolytes that generate a positive charge.

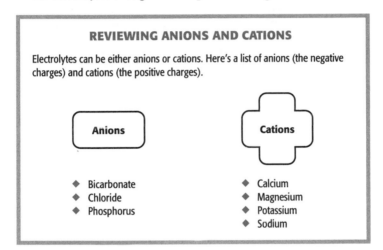

REVIEWING ANIONS AND CATIONS

Electrolytes can be either anions or cations. Here's a list of anions (the negative charges) and cations (the positive charges).

Anions

Cations

- ◆ Bicarbonate
- ◆ Chloride
- ◆ Phosphorus

- ◆ Calcium
- ◆ Magnesium
- ◆ Potassium
- ◆ Sodium

- Extracellular electrolytes exert their effects outside the cells.
- Sodium and chloride are the major electrolytes in extracellular fluid; calcium and bicarbonate are also extracellular electrolytes.

MAJOR EXTRACELLULAR ELECTROLYTES

- Sodium – helps nerve cells and muscle cells interact.
- Chloride – maintains osmotic pressure and helps gastric mucosal cells produce hydrochloric acid.

- Calcium – stabilizes cell membranes and reduces permeability, transmits nerve impulses, contracts muscles, coagulates blood, and forms bones and teeth.
- Bicarbonate – plays a role in acid-base balance.

◆ Intracellular electrolytes work inside the cells.
◆ Potassium, phosphate, and magnesium are the most plentiful
  intracellular electrolytes.

MAJOR INTRACELLULAR ELECTROLYTES

◆ Potassium – is responsible for cell excitability, nerve impulse conduction, resting membrane potential, muscle contraction, myocardial membrane responsiveness, and intracellular osmolality.

◆ Phosphate – is responsible for energy metabolism.

◆ Magnesium – is responsible for enzyme reactions, neuromuscular contractions, normal functioning of nervous and cardiovascular systems, protein synthesis, and sodium and potassium ion transportation.

Factors affecting electrolyte balance

◆ Fluid intake and output.
◆ Acid-base balance.
◆ Hormone secretion.
◆ Normal cell functioning.
◆ Normal organ and gland functioning.

ORGANS AND GLANDS IN ELECTROLYTE BALANCE

◆ Lungs and liver – regulate sodium and water balance and blood pressure.
◆ Heart – secretes atrial natriuretic peptide, causing sodium excretion.
◆ Sweat glands – excrete sodium, potassium, chloride, and water through sweat.
◆ GI tract – absorbs and excretes fluid and electrolytes.

◆ Parathyroid glands – secrete parathyroid hormone, which draws calcium into the blood and helps move phosphorus to the kidneys for excretion.
◆ Thyroid gland – secretes calcitonin, which prevents calcium release from the bone.

 AGE ALERT *An infant's immature kidneys can't reabsorb electrolytes as efficiently as an adult's kidneys can, so the infant is at a higher risk for electrolyte imbalances.*

Electrolyte levels

◆ Only extracellular (serum) electrolyte levels are measured.
◆ Electrolyte levels are reported in milliequivalents per liter
(mEq/L [SI, mmol/L]) or milligrams per deciliter (mg/dL [SI,
mmol/L]), a measure of the ion's chemical activity.

NORMAL ELECTROLYTE LEVELS

To maintain homeostasis, the body keeps electrolytes within a normal range, as
shown below. All normal electrolyte levels are measured in serum.

Electrolyte	Normal levels
Sodium	135 to 145 mEq/L (SI, 135 to 145 mmol/L)
Potassium	3.5 to 5 mEq/L (SI, 3.5 to 5 mmol/L)
Calcium, total	8.2 to 10.2 mg/dl (SI, 2.05 to 2.54 mmol/L)
Calcium, ionized	4.65 to 5.28 mg/dl (SI, 1.1 to 1.25 mmol/L)
Phosphates	2.7 to 4.5 mg/dl (SI, 0.87 to 1.45 mmol/L)
Magnesium	1.5 to 2.5 mEq/L (SI, 1.5 to 2.5 mmol/L)
Chloride	96 to 106 mEq/L (SI, 96 to 106 mmol/L)

Acid-base balance

◆ The chemical reactions that sustain life depend on a balance between acids and bases in the body.

◆ Acids consist of molecules that can give up hydrogen molecules to other molecules, as in solutions with a pH below 7 (SI, 7).

◆ Bases consist of molecules that can accept hydrogen molecules, as in solutions with a pH above 7 (SI, 7).

◆ To assess acid-base balance, you must know the pH of the blood.

◆ Normally, the pH ranges from 7.35 to 7.45 (SI, 7.35 to 7.45), which is slightly alkaline.

◆ A pH below 7.35 (SI, 7.35) is abnormally acidic; a pH above 7.45 (SI, 7.45) is abnormally alkaline.

DEVIATION FROM NORMAL pH

◆ Compromises well-being, electrolyte balance, activity of critical enzymes, muscle contraction, and basic cellular function.

◆ Is usually fatal if below 6.8 (SI, 6.8) or above 7.8 (SI, 7.8).

◆ Indicates alkalosis if above 7.45 (SI, 7.45).

◆ Indicates acidosis if below 7.35 (SI, 7.35).

Acid-base regulators

◆ When the pH rises or falls, three systems work to create acid-base balance.

◆ Chemical buffers instantly combine with the offending acid or base, neutralizing harmful effects until other regulators take over.

◆ The respiratory system uses hypoventilation and hyperventilation to regulate acid excretion or retention within minutes of a pH change.

◆ The kidneys excrete or retain more acids or bases as needed, restoring the normal balance within hours or days.

 AGE ALERT *An older adult's respiratory system may be compromised and less effective in regulating acid-base balance. Ammonia production decreases with age, and the kidneys of an older adult can't handle excess acid as well as the kidneys of a younger adult.*

ABG analysis

- ◆ Arterial blood gas (ABG) analysis can help you assess breathing effectiveness and acid-base balance.
- ◆ This test also helps monitor a patient's response to treatment.
- ◆ When interpreting ABG values, follow a consistent sequence to analyze the information.

Determine the pH

- ◆ Check the pH first because this figure forms the basis for understanding most other figures.
- ◆ If the pH is abnormal, determine whether it reflects acidosis (below 7.35 [SI, 7.35]) or alkalosis (above 7.45 [SI, 7.45]).
- ◆ Then figure out whether the cause is respiratory or metabolic.

NORMAL RANGES FOR KEY ABG VALUES

- ◆ pH – 7.35 to 7.45 (SI, 7.35 to 7.45)
- ◆ $Paco_2$ – 35 to 45 mm Hg (SI, 4.7 to 5.3 kPa)
- ◆ HCO_3^- – 22 to 25 mEq/L (SI, 22 to 25 mmol/L)

Determine the Paco$_2$

◆ Remember that the Paco$_2$ value provides information about the respiratory component of acid-base balance.

◆ If the Paco$_2$ is abnormal, determine whether it's low (less than 35 mm Hg [SI, 4.7 kPa]) or high (greater than 45 mm Hg [SI, 5.3 kPa]).

◆ Then determine whether the abnormal result corresponds with a change in the pH.

◆ If the pH is high, expect the Paco$_2$ to be low (hypocapnia), indicating that the problem is primarily respiratory in origin.

◆ If the pH is low, expect the Paco$_2$ to be high (hypercapnia), indicating that the problem is respiratory acidosis.

Watch the bicarbonate

◆ Examine the bicarbonate (HCO$_3$$^-$) level, which provides information about the metabolic aspect of acid-base balance.

◆ If the HCO$_3$$^-$ level is abnormal, determine whether it's low (less than 22 mEq/L [SI, 22 mmol/L]) or high (greater than 25 mEq/L [SI, 25 mmol/L]).

◆ Determine whether the abnormal result corresponds with the change in the pH.

◆ If the pH is high, expect the HCO$_3$$^-$ level to be high, indicating that the problem is primarily metabolic in origin.

◆ If the pH is low, expect the HCO$_3$$^-$ level to be low, indicating that the problem is metabolic acidosis.

Look for compensation

◆ Check for a change in the $Paco_2$ and HCO_3^- levels. One value indicates the primary source of the pH change; the other, the body's effort to compensate for the disturbance.

◆ Consider whether compensation is complete or partial.

◆ Complete compensation occurs when the body compensates so effectively that the pH falls within the normal range.

◆ Partial compensation occurs when the pH remains outside the normal range.

◆ Compensation involves opposites. For example, if results indicate primary metabolic acidosis, compensation will take the form of respiratory alkalosis.

Determine the Pao_2 and Sao_2

◆ Check the Pao_2 and Sao_2 values, which provide information about the patient's oxygenation.

◆ If the values are abnormal, determine whether they're high (Pao_2 greater than 100 mm Hg [SI, 13.3 kPa]) or low (Pao_2 less than 80 mm Hg [SI, 10.6 kPa] and Sao_2 less than 94% [SI, 0.94]).

◆ Consider the implications of your findings. Pao_2 reflects the body's ability to pick up oxygen from the lungs.

◆ A low Pao_2 value represents hypoxemia and can cause hyperventilation.

◆ The Pao_2 value also indicates when to make adjustments in the concentration of oxygen being given to a patient.

Avoid inaccurate ABG values

- To prevent inaccurate ABG values, be sure to use proper technique.
- Avoid delays in getting the sample to the laboratory.
- Don't draw blood for ABG analysis within 15 to 20 minutes of a procedure, such as suctioning or administering a respiratory treatment.
- Remove air bubbles from the syringe because they could affect the oxygen level.
- Don't get venous blood in the syringe because it could alter the carbon dioxide and oxygen levels and pH.

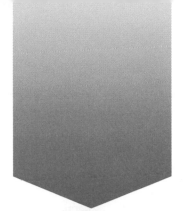

2

Fluid imbalances

A look at fluid imbalance

- ◆ When the body can't compensate for fluid deficits or excesses, an imbalance occurs.
- ◆ Fluid imbalances include dehydration, hypovolemia, hypervolemia, and water intoxication.
- ◆ Changes in fluid volume commonly affect the blood pressure, which makes it a critical assessment.
- ◆ Changes in fluid volume may also affect the pulmonary artery pressure (PAP), central venous pressure (CVP), pulmonary artery wedge pressure (PAWP), and cardiac output.

Dehydration

◆ The body constantly loses water, and a person responds by
  drinking fluids and consuming foods that contain water.
◆ If lost water isn't adequately replaced, the cells can lose water,
  which can lead to dehydration.

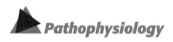*Pathophysiology*

WHAT HAPPENS IN DEHYDRATION

Body loses fluid.

Blood solute concentration (osmolality) increases.

Serum sodium level rises.

Water molecules shift out of cells into more concentrated blood.

Water intake and retention aren't sufficient to restore fluid volume.

Cells shrink as more fluid shifts out of them.

Patient develops mental status changes, which may lead to seizures and coma.

Causes

◆ Diabetes insipidus.
◆ Fever.
◆ Diarrhea.
◆ Renal failure.
◆ Hyperglycemia.

 AGE ALERT *Elderly and very young patients commonly develop fluid and electrolyte imbalances for similar reasons, such as:*

  – *inability to obtain fluid without help.*
  – *inability to express feelings of thirst.*
  – *inaccurate assessment of urine output.*
  – *loss of fluid caused by fever, diarrhea, or vomiting.*

Signs and symptoms

◆ Irritability and confusion.
◆ Dizziness.
◆ Weakness.
◆ Extreme thirst.
◆ Fever.
◆ Dry skin and mucous membranes.
◆ Sunken eyeballs.
◆ Poor skin turgor.
◆ Decreased urine output.
◆ Increased heart rate with decreased blood pressure.

Diagnostic test results

◆ Elevated hematocrit (HCT).
◆ Serum osmolality above 300 mOsm/kg (or 50 to 200 mOsm/kg in a patient with diabetes insipidus).
◆ Serum sodium level above 145 mEq/L (SI, 145 mmol/L).
◆ Urine specific gravity above 1.030 (or less than 1.005 in a patient with diabetes insipidus).

Management

- ◆ Encourage the patient to drink salt-free oral fluids if tolerated.
- ◆ Begin emergency treatment if your patient displays impaired mental status, seizures, or coma.
- ◆ Administer I.V. fluids to a severely dehydrated patient, using hypotonic, low-sodium solutions, such as dextrose 5% in water.
- ◆ Replace lost fluids gradually over 48 hours.
- ◆ Assess for signs and symptoms of cerebral edema, which can result from too-rapid administration of I.V. solutions.

SIGNS AND SYMPTOMS OF CEREBRAL EDEMA

- ◆ Headache
- ◆ Confusion
- ◆ Irritability
- ◆ Lethargy

- ◆ Nausea and vomiting
- ◆ Widening pulse pressure
- ◆ Decreasing pulse rate
- ◆ Seizures

- ◆ Administer vasopressin (Pitressin) to a patient with diabetes insipidus if prescribed.
- ◆ Assess for complications of concentrated vascular volume, including thrombophlebitis and pulmonary emboli.
- ◆ Assess for diaphoresis, which can be a major source of water loss.
- ◆ Monitor the sodium level, urine osmolality, and urine specific gravity.

Hypervolemia

◆ Hypervolemia is an excess of isotonic fluid (water and sodium) in the extracellular (interstitial or intravascular) compartment.
◆ This fluid imbalance doesn't usually affect osmolality because fluid and solutes are gained in equal proportions.
◆ With mild to moderate hypervolemia, the patient's weight may increase 5% to 10%; with severe hypervolemia, it may increase more than 10%.
◆ Elderly patients and patients with impaired renal or cardiovascular function are most susceptible to hypervolemia.

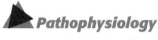 *Pathophysiology*

WHAT HAPPENS IN HYPERVOLEMIA

Excess sodium or fluid is consumed or retained.

⬇

Fluid moves out of blood vessels into the interstitial space.

⬇

Extracellular fluid accumulates in the interstitial or intravascular compartment.

⬇

Edema develops in the lungs and other tissues.

Causes

- ◆ Excess sodium or fluid intake.
  - – I.V. administration of normal saline or lactated Ringer's solution.
  - – Blood or plasma replacement.
  - – High intake of dietary sodium.
- ◆ Fluid and sodium retention.
  - – Heart failure.
  - – Cirrhosis.
  - – Nephrotic syndrome.
  - – Corticosteroid use.
  - – Hyperaldosteronism.
  - – Low intake of dietary protein.
- ◆ Fluid shift into the intravascular space.
  - – Fluid movement after burn treatment.
  - – I.V. administration of hypertonic fluid.
  - – Use of albumin or other plasma proteins.

Signs and symptoms

- ◆ Tachypnea and dyspnea.
- ◆ Crackles.
- ◆ Rapid, bounding pulse.
- ◆ Hypertension (unless the heart is failing).
- ◆ Increased CVP, PAP, and PAWP.
- ◆ Distended neck and hand veins.
- ◆ Acute weight gain.
- ◆ Peripheral edema.
- ◆ S_3 gallop.
- ◆ Pulmonary edema (with prolonged hypervolemia).

EVALUATING PITTING EDEMA

You can evaluate edema using a scale of +1 to +4. Press your fingertip firmly into the skin over a bony surface for a few seconds. Then note the depth of the imprint your finger leaves on the skin.

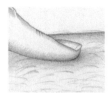 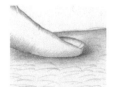 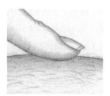

A slight imprint indicates +1 pitting edema.

A deep imprint, with the skin slow to return to its original contour, indicates +4 pitting edema.

When the skin resists pressure but appears distended, the condition is called brawny edema. In brawny edema, the skin swells so much that fluid can't be displaced.

HOW PULMONARY EDEMA DEVELOPS

Excess fluid volume that lasts a long time can cause pulmonary edema. The illustrations here show how that process occurs.

Normal

Normal pulmonary fluid movement depends on the equal force of two opposing pressures – hydrostatic pressure and plasma oncotic pressure from protein molecules in the blood.

Congestion

Abnormally high pulmonary hydrostatic pressure (indicated by increased pulmonary artery wedge pressure) forces fluid out of the capillaries and into the interstitial space, causing pulmonary congestion.

Edema

When the amount of interstitial fluid becomes excessive, fluid is forced into the alveoli. Pulmonary edema results. Fluid fills the alveoli and prevents the exchange of gases.

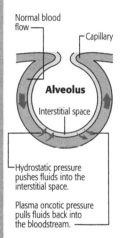

Normal blood flow

Capillary

Alveolus

Interstitial space

Hydrostatic pressure pushes fluids into the interstitial space.

Plasma oncotic pressure pulls fluids back into the bloodstream.

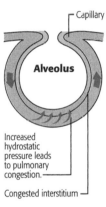

Capillary

Alveolus

Increased hydrostatic pressure leads to pulmonary congestion.

Congested interstitium

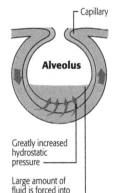

Capillary

Alveolus

Greatly increased hydrostatic pressure

Large amount of fluid is forced into the alveolus.

Diagnostic test results

◆ Low HCT because of hemodilution.
◆ Normal serum sodium level.
◆ Lower serum potassium and blood urea nitrogen (BUN) levels because of hemodilution (or higher levels in a patient with renal failure or impaired renal perfusion).
◆ Low oxygen level.
◆ Pulmonary congestion on chest X-rays.

 ### *Management*

◆ Restrict the patient's sodium and fluid intake.
◆ Administer diuretics as prescribed.
◆ Provide oxygen therapy.
◆ Treat heart failure with digoxin (Lanoxin) and bedrest.
◆ Treat pulmonary edema with drugs that dilate blood vessels, such as morphine (Roxanol) and nitroglycerin (Nitro-Bid).
◆ If the patient has renal failure and diuretics aren't effective, provide hemodialysis or another form of dialysis.
◆ Assess for signs and symptoms of hypovolemia, which can result from overcorrection of hypervolemia.
◆ Monitor the results of arterial blood gas analysis to detect changes in oxygenation and acid-base balance.
◆ Monitor the potassium level, which typically decreases with diuretic use and increases with renal failure.
◆ Assess for an S_3 heart sound that's heard when the ventricles are volume overloaded.

Hypovolemia

◆ Hypovolemia refers to an isotonic fluid loss — including the loss of fluids and solutes — from the extracellular space.
◆ If hypovolemia isn't detected early and treated, it may progress to hypovolemic shock.

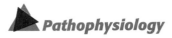 *Pathophysiology*

WHAT HAPPENS IN HYPOVOLEMIA WITH THIRD-SPACE SHIFTING

Capillary membrane permeability increases or plasma colloid osmotic pressure decreases.

Fluid moves out of the intravascular space.
Fluid shifts into the abdominal cavity, pleural cavity, or pericardial sac.

Reduced fluid intake may exacerbate the fluid shift.

Patient displays weight loss, mental status changes, and orthostatic hypotension.

Causes

- ◆ Excessive fluid loss.
  - – Abdominal surgery.
  - – Diabetes mellitus (from polyuria).
  - – Diarrhea.
  - – Excessive diuretic therapy.
  - – Excessive laxative use.
  - – Excessive sweating.
  - – Fever.
  - – Fistulas.
  - – Hemorrhage.
  - – Nasogastric (NG) drainage.
  - – Renal failure with polyuria.
  - – Vomiting.
- ◆ Third-space shifting.
  - – Acute intestinal obstruction.
  - – Acute peritonitis.
  - – Burns (in the initial phase).
  - – Crush injuries.
  - – Hip fracture.
  - – Hypoalbuminemia.
  - – Pleural effusion.

Signs and symptoms

◆ Altered mental status.
◆ Tachycardia.
◆ Orthostatic hypotension followed by marked hypotension.
◆ Decreased urine output (10 to 30 ml/hour).
◆ Weight loss.
◆ Cool, pale skin over arms and legs.
◆ Delayed capillary refill.
◆ Thirst.
◆ Flat jugular veins.
◆ Decreased CVP.

Diagnostic test results

◆ Decreased hemoglobin level and HCT, with hemorrhage.
◆ Elevated BUN level.
◆ Increased urine specific gravity, with the kidneys trying to conserve fluid.
◆ Normal or high serum sodium level (above 145 mEq/L [SI, 145 mmol/L]), depending on the amount of fluid and sodium lost.

Management

◆ Replace lost fluids with isotonic solutions (fluids of the same concentration).

◆ Administer I.V. fluids in a fluid challenge, giving them in large amounts over a short time. Use short, large-bore catheters for rapid infusion.

◆ Provide numerous I.V. infusions for hypovolemic shock.

◆ Administer oxygen.

◆ Lower the head of the bed or elevate the foot of the bed to increase cerebral perfusion.

◆ Administer a vasopressor, such as dopamine (Intropin), to raise the blood pressure.

◆ Administer blood transfusions if the patient is hemorrhaging.

◆ Monitor hemodynamic values (CVP, PAP, PAWP, and cardiac output) to assess the patient's response to treatment.

◆ Monitor for signs and symptoms of fluid overload, such as crackles, which may result from aggressive fluid replacement.

◆ Closely monitor the patient's mental status and vital signs, staying alert for blood pressure changes and arrhythmias.

Water intoxication

◆ Water intoxication occurs when excess fluid moves from the extracellular space to the intracellular space.

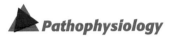 *Pathophysiology*

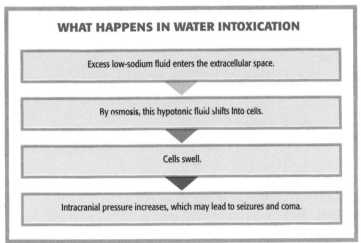

WHAT HAPPENS IN WATER INTOXICATION

Excess low-sodium fluid enters the extracellular space.

By osmosis, this hypotonic fluid shifts into cells.

Cells swell.

Intracranial pressure increases, which may lead to seizures and coma.

Causes

◆ Syndrome of inappropriate antidiuretic hormone secretion.
◆ Rapid infusion of a hypotonic solution.
◆ Excessive use of tap water as an NG tube irrigant or enema.
◆ Psychogenic polydipsia.

Signs and symptoms

◆ Increased intracranial pressure.
◆ Muscle cramps and weakness.
◆ Nausea and vomiting.
◆ Headache.
◆ Changes in personality, behavior, and level of consciousness.
◆ Twitching.
◆ Thirst.
◆ Dyspnea on exertion.
◆ Bradycardia and widened pulse pressure.

Diagnostic test results

◆ Serum osmolality below 280 mOsm/kg.
◆ Serum sodium level below 125 mEq/L (SI, 125 mmol/L).

Management

◆ Correct the underlying cause. For example, slow or temporarily discontinue a hypotonic solution infusion; or replace tap water with sterile water or a hypertonic solution for NG tube irrigation or enemas.
◆ Restrict oral and parenteral fluid intake and avoid the use of hypotonic I.V. solutions until the serum sodium level rises.
◆ Administer a hypertonic I.V. solution slowly, using an infusion pump.
◆ Monitor the patient's neurologic status, staying alert for deterioration.
◆ Monitor the serum sodium level.
◆ Institute seizure precautions as needed.

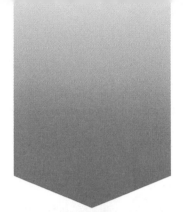

3

Electrolyte imbalances

Hypernatremia

◆ Hypernatremia is characterized by a serum sodium level above 145 mEq/L (SI, 145 mmol/L).
◆ In hypernatremia, the body has an excess of sodium relative to water.
◆ Severe hypernatremia can lead to seizures, coma, and permanent neurologic damage.
◆ Water deficit or excess sodium intake can lead to hypernatremia, making body fluids more hypertonic (more concentrated).

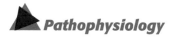 *Pathophysiology*

WHAT HAPPENS IN HYPERNATREMIA

Sodium intake or water loss becomes excessive.

▼

Serum osmolality increases.

▼

Fluid moves by osmosis from inside cells to outside cells to balance intracellular and extracellular fluid levels.

▼

Cells become dehydrated, causing neurologic impairment; extracellular fluid volume in vessels increases, causing hypervolemia.

Causes

◆ Water deficit.
  – Fever.
  – Heat stroke.
  – Pulmonary infections.
  – Extensive burns.
  – Severe diarrhea.
  – Hyperosmolar hyperglycemic nonketotic syndrome.
  – Urea diuresis.
  – Diabetes insipidus.

 AGE ALERT *Infants and children are at greater risk for hypernatremia because they tend to lose more water as a result of diarrhea, vomiting, inadequate fluid intake, and fever.*

◆ Excess sodium intake.
  – Overconsumption of dietary sodium.
  – Use of certain drugs.
  – Near drowning in salt water.
  – Cushing's syndrome.
  – Hyperaldosteronism.

DRUGS THAT CAN CAUSE HYPERNATREMIA

◆ Antacids with sodium bicarbonate (Citrocarbonate)
◆ Antibiotics such as ticarcillin disodium-clavulanate potassium (Timentin)
◆ Salt tablets
◆ Sodium bicarbonate injections such as those given during cardiac arrest
◆ I.V. sodium chloride preparations
◆ Sodium polystyrene sulfonate (Kayexalate)

Signs and symptoms

◆ Agitation and restlessness.
◆ Confusion.
◆ Flushed skin.
◆ Intense thirst.
◆ Lethargy.
◆ Low-grade fever.
◆ Signs and symptoms of hypervolemia (from sodium gain), such as bounding pulses, dyspnea, and hypertension.
◆ Signs and symptoms of hypovolemia (from water loss), such as dry mucous membranes, oliguria, and orthostatic hypotension.
◆ Twitching.
◆ Weakness.

Diagnostic test results

◆ Serum osmolality above 300 mOsm/kg.
◆ Serum sodium level above 145 mEq/L (SI, 145 mmol/L).
◆ Urine specific gravity above 1.030 (or less than 1.005 in a patient with diabetes insipidus).

Management

- Individualize treatment based on the cause of hypernatremia.
- Replace oral fluids gradually over 48 hours to avoid shifting water into brain cells.

 ALERT *If too much water is replaced too quickly, water moves into brain cells and they swell, causing cerebral edema.*

- Replace fluids with a salt-free I.V. solution such as dextrose 5% in water. Use an infusion pump to help prevent cerebral edema.
- Then infuse half-normal saline solution to prevent hyponatremia and cerebral edema.
- Restrict the patient's sodium intake.
- Administer a diuretic along with oral or I.V. fluids.
- Frequently check the patient's neurologic status.
- Monitor the serum sodium level.
- Monitor urine specific gravity.
- Monitor fluid intake and output and daily weight measurements.

Hyponatremia

◆ Hyponatremia is characterized by a serum sodium level below 135 mEq/L (SI, 135 mmol/L).
◆ In hyponatremia, body fluids are diluted and cells swell from decreased extracellular fluid osmolality.
◆ Severe hyponatremia (sodium level below 110 mEq/L [SI, 110 mmol/L]) can lead to seizures, coma, and permanent neurologic damage.
◆ Hyponatremia can be triggered by sodium loss, water gain (dilutional hyponatremia), or inadequate sodium intake (depletional hyponatremia).
◆ Hyponatremia can be hypovolemic (with decreased extracellular fluid volume), hypervolemic (with increased extracellular fluid volume), or isovolumic (with extracellular fluid volume equal to intracellular fluid volume).

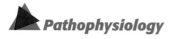 *Pathophysiology*

WHAT HAPPENS IN HYPONATREMIA

Sodium loss or water gain increases, or sodium intake decreases.

Fluid moves by osmosis from the extracellular space (which has more water and less sodium) into the more concentrated intracellular space.

Cells contain more fluid, and blood vessels contain less.
Cerebral edema and hypovolemia can occur.

Causes

- ◆ Hypovolemic hyponatremia.
  - Osmotic diuresis.
  - Salt-losing nephritis.
  - Adrenal insufficiency.
  - Diuretic use.
  - Vomiting.
  - Diarrhea.
  - Fistulas.
  - Gastric suctioning.
  - Excessive diaphoresis.
  - Cystic fibrosis.
  - Burns.
  - Wound drainage.
- ◆ Hypervolemic hyponatremia.
  - Heart or liver failure.
  - Nephrotic syndrome.
  - Excessive use of hypotonic fluids.
  - Hyperaldosteronism.
- ◆ Isovolumic hyponatremia.
  - Glucocorticoid deficiency.
  - Hypothyroidism.
  - Renal failure.
  - Syndrome of inappropriate antidiuretic hormone (SIADH) secretion.

DRUGS THAT CAN CAUSE HYPONATREMIA

Anticonvulsants
- Carbamazepine (Tegretol)

Antidiabetics
- Chlorpropamide (Diabinese)
- Tolbutamide (Orinase), rarely

Antineoplastics
- Cyclophosphamide (Cytoxan)
- Vincristine (Oncovin)

Antipsychotics
- Fluphenazine (Prolixin)
- Thioridazine (Mellaril)
- Thiothixene (Navane)

Diuretics
- Bumetanide (Bumex)
- Ethacrynic acid (Edecrin)
- Furosemide (Lasix)
- Thiazides, such as chlorothiazide (Diuril) and hydrochlorothiazide (HydroDIURIL)

Sedatives
- Barbiturates, such as phenobarbital (Luminal) and secobarbital (Seconal)
- Morphine (Roxanol)

Signs and symptoms

- ◆ Abdominal cramps.
- ◆ Altered level of consciousness (LOC), such as lethargy and confusion.
- ◆ Headache.
- ◆ Muscle twitching, tremors, and weakness.
- ◆ Nausea.
- ◆ Seizures.

Hyponatremia caused by hypovolemia

- ◆ Dry mucous membranes.
- ◆ Orthostatic hypotension or low blood pressure.
- ◆ Poor skin turgor.
- ◆ Tachycardia.
- ◆ Weak pulses.

Hyponatremia caused by hypervolemia

- ◆ Edema.
- ◆ Hypertension.
- ◆ Rapid, bounding pulses.
- ◆ Weight gain.

Diagnostic test results

◆ Elevated hematocrit and plasma protein levels.
◆ Serum osmolality below 280 mOsm/kg (dilute blood).
◆ Serum sodium level below 135 mEq/L (SI, 135 mmol/L).
◆ Urine specific gravity below 1.010 (or increased urine specific gravity and urine sodium level in a patient with SIADH secretion).

 Management

Mild hyponatremia with hypervolemia or isovolumia

◆ Restrict the patient's fluid intake.
◆ Provide oral sodium supplements.

Mild hyponatremia with hypovolemia

◆ Administer isotonic I.V. fluids, such as normal saline solution, to restore volume.
◆ Provide high-sodium foods.

Severe hyponatremia

◆ Infuse a hypertonic solution, such as 3% or 5% saline solution, giving it slowly and in small volumes to prevent fluid overload.
◆ Watch for signs and symptoms of circulatory overload or worsening neurologic status.

 ALERT *Hypervolemic patients shouldn't receive hypertonic sodium chloride solutions, except in rare instances of severe symptomatic hyponatremia.*

◆ Monitor the serum sodium level to evaluate the patient's response to therapy.
◆ Monitor the patient's fluid intake and output and daily weight measurements.

Hyperkalemia

- ◆ Hyperkalemia is characterized by a serum potassium level above 5 mEq/L (SI, 5 mmol/L).
- ◆ In hyperkalemia, the body has an excess of potassium relative to water.
- ◆ Hyperkalemia is the most dangerous electrolyte disorder. Even a slight increase in the potassium level can profoundly affect the neuromuscular and cardiovascular systems.
- ◆ This electrolyte imbalance can result from increased potassium intake, decreased potassium excretion, or cellular injury that causes potassium release from cells.

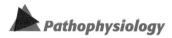 *Pathophysiology*

WHAT HAPPENS IN HYPERKALEMIA

Potassium intake increases, or potassium excretion decreases.

▼

Potassium shifts out of cells into extracellular fluid.

▼

Extracellular potassium level rises.

▼

Patient develops neuromuscular and cardiac signs and symptoms.

Causes

◆ Increased potassium intake.
 – Overconsumption of dietary potassium.
 – Excessive use of salt substitutes or potassium supplements.
 – High-volume blood transfusion.
 – Use of certain drugs.
◆ Decreased potassium excretion.
 – Acute or chronic renal failure.
 – Disorders that damage the kidneys.
 – Addison's disease.
 – Hypoaldosteronism.
◆ Potassium release from cells.
 – Burns.
 – Severe infection.
 – Trauma.
 – Crush injury.
 – Intravascular hemolysis.
 – Metabolic acidosis.
 – Insulin deficiency.

DRUGS THAT CAN CAUSE HYPERKALEMIA

◆ Angiotensin-converting enzyme inhibitors
◆ Antibiotics
◆ Beta-adrenergic blockers
◆ Chemotherapeutic drugs
◆ Nonsteroidal anti-inflammatory drugs
◆ Potassium, in excessive amounts
◆ Spironolactone (Aldactone)

Signs and symptoms

◆ Abdominal cramps.
◆ Decreased heart rate.
◆ Diarrhea.
◆ Hypotension.
◆ Irregular pulse rate.
◆ Irritability.
◆ Muscle weakness, especially in the legs.
◆ Nausea.
◆ Paresthesia.

Diagnostic test results

◆ Decreased arterial pH, indicating acidosis.
◆ Electrocardiogram (ECG) changes, especially tall, tented T waves and possibly flattened P waves, prolonged PR intervals, widened QRS complexes, and depressed ST segments.
◆ Serum potassium level above 5 mEq/L (SI, 5 mmol/L).

Management

◆ Restrict the patient's potassium intake.
◆ Stop or readjust drugs that may be contributing to hyper-kalemia.
◆ Treat mild cases with a loop diuretic, such as furosemide (Lasix).

 ALERT *For a patient with renal failure, diuretics may not be effective. If so, plan to use hemodialysis or similar therapy to lower the potassium level.*

◆ Administer sodium polystyrene sulfonate (Kayexalate) by mouth, via nasogastric (NG) tube, or as a retention enema. Give this drug with sorbitol or another osmotic substance to promote its excretion.
◆ Closely monitor the patient's cardiac status, including ECG trac-ings.
◆ Administer 10% calcium gluconate to counteract the myocardial effects of hyperkalemia.
◆ Administer regular insulin and hypertonic dextrose by I.V. to move potassium into the cells. During therapy, monitor for hy-poglycemia.
◆ Administer sodium bicarbonate to a patient with acidosis to shift potassium into the cells.
◆ Closely monitor the patient's fluid intake and output.
◆ If the patient doesn't respond to treatment, prepare him for di-alysis.

Hypokalemia

- Hypokalemia is characterized by a serum potassium level below 3.5 mEq/L (SI, 3.5 mmol/L).
- In hypokalemia, potassium deficiency occurs because the body can't effectively conserve potassium.
- Hypokalemia can result from inadequate potassium intake or excessive potassium output.

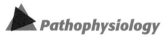 *Pathophysiology*

WHAT HAPPENS IN HYPOKALEMIA

Potassium intake decreases, or potassium loss increases.

Potassium shifts from extracellular fluid to intracellular fluid.

Intracellular potassium level rises.

Cells can't function properly.

Muscular, GI, and cardiac dysfunctions occur.

Causes

◆ Inadequate potassium intake.
  – Low consumption of potassium-rich foods.
  – Use of potassium-deficient I.V. fluids.
◆ Excessive potassium output.
  – Severe GI fluid loss (as with suction, lavage, prolonged vomiting, or diarrhea).
  – Severe diaphoresis.
  – Diuresis (as with recent kidney transplantation or a high urine glucose level).
  – Use of certain drugs.
  – Renal tubular acidosis.
  – Magnesium depletion.
  – Cushing's syndrome.
  – Stress.

DRUGS THAT CAN CAUSE HYPOKALEMIA

◆ Adrenergics, such as albuterol (Ventolin) and epinephrine (Primatene)
◆ Antibiotics, such as amphotericin B (Amphotec), carbenicillin (Geocillin), and gentamicin (Garamycin)

◆ Cisplatin (Platinol-AQ)
◆ Corticosteroids
◆ Diuretics, such as furosemide (Lasix) and thiazides
◆ Insulin (Humulin, Novolin)
◆ Laxatives, with excessive use

Signs and symptoms

◆ Anorexia.
◆ Constipation.
◆ Hyporeflexia.
◆ Muscle cramps and weakness.
◆ Nausea and vomiting.
◆ Orthostatic hypotension.
◆ Paresthesia.
◆ Polyuria.
◆ Weak, irregular pulses.

Diagnostic test results

◆ Elevated pH and bicarbonate levels.
◆ ECG changes, such as flattened T waves, depressed ST segments, and characteristic U waves.
◆ Serum potassium level below 3.5 mEq/L (SI, 3.5 mmol/L).
◆ Slightly elevated serum glucose level.

Management

- Focus treatment on restoring potassium balance, removing the underlying cause, and preventing complications, such as arrhythmias, cardiac arrest, and respiratory arrest.
- Place the patient on a high-potassium diet.
- Provide oral potassium supplements as needed.
- To prevent gastric irritation from oral potassium supplements, administer them in at least 4 oz (118 ml) of fluid or with food.

  ALERT *To prevent a quick load of potassium from entering the body, don't crush slow-release potassium tablets.*

- If the patient can't tolerate oral potassium supplements or has severe hypokalemia, administer I.V. potassium, using an infusion pump to control the flow rate.

  ALERT *Never give potassium by I.V. push or bolus because such rapid administration could be fatal.*

- When selecting a vein for I.V. therapy, remember that potassium preparations can irritate peripheral veins and cause discomfort. When possible, choose a more proximal site, such as an antecubital vein rather than a vein in the hand.
- Consider switching the patient to a potassium-sparing diuretic if indicated.
- Monitor the patient's vital signs, particularly noting orthostatic hypotension.
- Monitor the heart rate and rhythm if the patient's potassium level is less than 3 mEq/L (SI, 3 mmol/L) or if the I.V. potassium infusion exceeds 5 mEq/hour (SI, 5 mmol/h).
- Assess the patient's respiratory status because hypokalemia can weaken or paralyze respiratory muscles. Keep a manual resuscitation bag at the bedside.

Hypermagnesemia

◆ Hypermagnesemia is characterized by a serum magnesium level above 2.1 mg/dl (SI, 1.05 mmol/L).

 AGE ALERT *Magnesium levels in pediatric patients differ from those in adults. In newborns, the normal magnesium level ranges from 1.5 to 2.2 mg/dl (SI, 0.62 to 0.91 mmol/L); in children, from 1.7 to 2.1 mg/dl (SI, 0.70 to 0.86 mmol/L).*

◆ In hypermagnesemia, the magnesium imbalance can result from impaired magnesium excretion or excessive magnesium intake.

 Pathophysiology

WHAT HAPPENS IN HYPERMAGNESEMIA

Magnesium excretion decreases, or magnesium intake increases.

▼

High magnesium level suppresses acetylcholine release at myoneural junctions.

▼

Reduced acetylcholine blocks neuromuscular transmission and reduces cell excitability.

▼

The neuromuscular and central nervous systems become depressed.

▼

Level of consciousness decreases and respiratory distress occurs.

▼

Arrhythmias and other cardiac complications may develop.

Causes

◆ Impaired magnesium excretion.
  – Renal dysfunction.
  – Advanced age.
  – Renal failure.
  – Addison's disease.
  – Adrenocortical insufficiency.
  – Diabetic ketoacidosis (DKA).
◆ Excessive magnesium intake.
  – Use of certain drugs.
  – Use of magnesium-rich dialysate for hemodialysis.
  – Use of magnesium-rich solutions for total parenteral nutrition (TPN).
  – Treatment with continuous infusion of magnesium sulfate.

DRUGS THAT CAN CAUSE HYPERMAGNESEMIA

◆ Antacids such as magnesium-aluminum combination drugs (Di-Gel, Gaviscon, Maalox)
◆ Laxatives that contain magnesium (Haley's M-O, magnesium citrate, Milk of Magnesia)

◆ Magnesium supplements, such as magnesium oxide (Mag-Ox 400) and magnesium sulfate

---

Signs and symptoms

◆ Bradycardia, possibly leading to heart block and cardiac arrest.
◆ Decreased LOC, progressing from drowsiness and lethargy to coma.
◆ Decreased muscle and nerve activity.
◆ Flushed skin and feelings of warmth.
◆ Hypoactive deep tendon reflexes (DTRs).
◆ Hypotension.
◆ Generalized weakness.
◆ Nausea and vomiting.
◆ Respirations that are slow, shallow, and depressed.
◆ Respiratory arrest.

Diagnostic test results

◆ ECG changes, such as prolonged PR intervals, widened QRS complexes, and tall T waves.

◆ Serum magnesium level above 2.6 mEq/L (SI, 1.07 mmol/L).

 ## *Management*

◆ If the patient has normal renal function, administer oral or I.V. fluids to rid the body of excessive magnesium.

◆ If fluid administration isn't effective, give a loop diuretic, such as furosemide (Lasix) to promote magnesium excretion.

◆ In an emergency, administer calcium gluconate (a magnesium antagonist).

◆ Provide mechanical ventilation if hypermagnesemia compromises respiratory function.

◆ For a patient with severe renal dysfunction, prepare for hemodialysis with a magnesium-free dialysate solution.

◆ Assess the patient's DTRs and muscle strength. Also assess his skin for flushing and diaphoresis.

◆ Closely monitor the patient's respiratory status.

◆ Monitor for fluid overload if the patient receives large volumes of fluid.

◆ Avoid the use of drugs that contain magnesium, and restrict the patient's dietary intake of magnesium.

◆ Closely monitor the patient receiving magnesium sulfate. Also monitor the newborn of a mother who received magnesium sulfate for hypertension or pre-term labor.

Hypomagnesemia

◆ Hypomagnesemia is characterized by a serum magnesium level below 1.3 mg/dl (SI, 0.65 mmol/L).

◆ This relatively common condition can lead to respiratory muscle paralysis, complete heart block, and coma.

◆ Hypomagnesemia can result from inadequate dietary intake of magnesium, inadequate magnesium absorption by the GI tract, or excessive magnesium loss from the GI or urinary tracts.

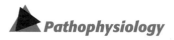 *Pathophysiology*

WHAT HAPPENS IN HYPOMAGNESEMIA

Magnesium intake or absorption decreases, or magnesium loss increases.

Magnesium moves out of cells to compensate for low extracellular magnesium level.

Cells become starved for magnesium.

Skeletal muscles weaken, and nerves and muscles become hyperirritable.

Causes

◆ Inadequate magnesium intake.
  - Chronic alcoholism.
  - Prolonged I.V. fluid therapy.
  - Use of TPN or enteral feeding formulas without sufficient magnesium.
◆ Inadequate GI absorption of magnesium.
  - Malabsorption syndrome.
  - Steatorrhea.
  - Ulcerative colitis.
  - Crohn's disease.
  - Bowel resection or similar GI surgery.
  - Cancer.
  - Pancreatic insufficiency.
  - Excess calcium or phosphorus in the GI tract.
◆ Excessive GI loss of magnesium.
  - Prolonged diarrhea.
  - Fistula drainage.
  - Laxative abuse.
  - NG tube suctioning.
  - Acute pancreatitis.
◆ Excessive urinary loss of magnesium.
  - Primary aldosteronism.
  - Hyperparathyroidism or hypoparathyroidism.
  - DKA.
  - Use of certain drugs.
  - Renal disorders, such as glomerulonephritis, pyelonephritis, and renal tubular acidosis.

DRUGS THAT CAN CAUSE HYPOMAGNESEMIA

- Aminoglycoside antibiotics, such as amikacin (Amikin), gentamicin (Garamycin), streptomycin (Streptomycin), and tobramycin (Nebcin)
- Amphotericin B (Fungizone)
- Cisplatin (Platinol-AQ)
- Cyclosporine (Sandimmune)
- Insulin (Humulin, Novolin)
- Laxatives
- Loop diuretics, such as bumetanide (Bumex), furosemide (Lasix), and torsemide (Demadex)
- Pentamidine isethionate (Nebu-Pent)
- Thiazide diuretics, such as chlorothiazide (Diuril) and hydrochlorothiazide (Hydro-DIURIL)

Signs and symptoms

- Altered LOC and confusion, hallucinations, or seizures.
- Anorexia and dysphagia.
- Arrhythmias, such as atrial fibrillation, heart block, paroxysmal atrial tachycardia, premature ventricular contractions, supraventricular tachycardia, torsades de pointes, ventricular fibrillation, and ventricular tachycardia.
- Chvostek's sign and Trousseau's sign.
- Hyperactive DTRs.
- Hypertension.
- Leg and foot cramps.
- Muscle weakness, twitching, tremors, or tetany.
- Nausea and vomiting.
- Respiratory difficulties.

Diagnostic test results

- ECG changes, such as prolonged PR intervals, widened QRS complexes, prolonged QT intervals, depressed ST segments, broad flattened T waves, and prominent U waves.
- Elevated serum digoxin level in a patient receiving the drug.
- Serum magnesium level below 1.3 mg/dl (SI, 0.65 mmol/L), possibly with a below-normal serum albumin level.
- Other electrolyte abnormalities, such as a below-normal serum potassium or calcium level.

Management

- Manage a mild deficiency with increased intake of magnesium-rich foods or with oral supplements. Continue oral magnesium replacement for several days after the serum magnesium level returns to normal.
- Treat a severe deficiency with I.V. or deep I.M. injections of magnesium sulfate.

   ALERT *Before administering magnesium, assess the patient's renal function. If renal function is impaired (urine output below 10 ml in 4 hours), monitor the magnesium level closely because this electrolyte is excreted by the kidneys.*

- Monitor the patient's neuromuscular status to detect hyperactive DTRs, tremors, and tetany.
- Check for Chvostek's and Trousseau's signs.
- Assess for dysphagia before giving the patient food.
- Monitor the patient's respiratory status, which can be compromised by hypomagnesemia-induced laryngeal stridor and breathing difficulty.
- Regularly assess the patient's urine output.
- If the patient receives digoxin (Lanoxin), monitor for signs and symptoms of digoxin toxicity because hypomagnesemia can increase the risk of this adverse reaction.
- Monitor all electrolyte levels because hypocalcemia and hypokalemia can cause hypomagnesemia, especially if the patient receives a diuretic.
- Institute seizure precautions as needed.

Hypercalcemia

◆ Hypercalcemia is characterized by a total serum calcium level above 10.2 mg/dl (SI, 2.54 mmol/L) and an ionized serum calcium level above 5.28 mg/dl (SI, 1.25 mmol/L).

◆ In hypercalcemia, the rate of calcium entry into extracellular fluid exceeds the rate of calcium excretion by the kidneys.

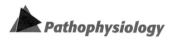 *Pathophysiology*

WHAT HAPPENS IN HYPERCALCEMIA

Calcium resorption from bone increases.

⬇

Calcium enters extracellular fluid at an increased rate.

⬇

Calcium movement into extracellular fluid exceeds the rate of calcium excretion by the kidneys.

⬇

Excess calcium enters cells.

⬇

Excess intracellular calcium decreases cell membrane excitability.

⬇

Reduced membrane excitability affects skeletal and cardiac muscles and the nervous system.

⬇

Patient may display fatigue, confusion, and decreased level of consciousness.

AGE ALERT *Pediatric patients normally have higher serum calcium levels than adults do. In fact, their serum calcium levels can rise as high as 11.2 mg/dl (SI, 2.79 mmol/L) during periods of increased bone growth. Geriatric patients normally have a narrower range of normal calcium levels than younger adults do. For older men, the range is 2.3 to 3.7 mg/dl (SI, 0.57 to 0.92 mmol/L); for older women, it's 2.8 to 4.1 mg/dl (SI, 0.25 to 1.02 mmol/L).*

Causes

◆ Increased calcium resorption from bone.
  – Hyperparathyroidism.
  – Cancer.
◆ Use of certain drugs.
◆ Increased calcium absorption or decreased calcium excretion.
  – Hyperthyroidism.
  – Multiple fractures.
  – Prolonged immobilization.
  – Hypophosphatemia.
  – Acidosis.

DRUGS THAT CAN CAUSE HYPERCALCEMIA

◆ Antacids that contain calcium (Tums)
◆ Calcium preparations (oral or I.V.)
◆ Lithium (Eskalith)
◆ Thiazide diuretics, such as chlorothiazide (Diuril) and hydrochlorothiazide (Hydro-DIURIL)
◆ Vitamin A (Aquasol A)
◆ Vitamin D (Calcijex)

Signs and symptoms

◆ Abdominal pain and constipation.
◆ Anorexia.
◆ Behavioral changes, including confusion.
◆ Bone pain.
◆ Decreased LOC, which may progress from lethargy to coma.
◆ Extreme thirst and polyuria.
◆ Hypertension.
◆ Hypoactive DTRs.
◆ Muscle weakness.
◆ Nausea and vomiting.

Diagnostic test results

◆ ECG changes, such as shortened QT intervals and shortened ST segments.
◆ Elevated serum digoxin level in a patient receiving the drug.
◆ Ionized calcium level above 5.28 mg/dl (SI, 1.25 mmol/L).
◆ Total serum calcium level above 10.2 mg/dl (SI, 2.54 mmol/L).
◆ X-rays revealing pathologic fractures.

Management

- Limit the patient's dietary calcium intake and discontinue drugs or infusions that contain calcium.
- Hydrate the patient with normal saline solution to promote diuresis and calcium excretion.
- Administer a loop diuretic such as furosemide (Lasix) to help promote calcium excretion.

     ALERT *Don't give a thiazide diuretic to a patient with hypercalcemia because it can inhibit calcium excretion.*

- For a patient with life-threatening hypercalcemia, prepare for dialysis.
- Administer a corticosteroid as prescribed to block bone resorption and decrease GI absorption of calcium.
- Give etidronate disodium (Didronel) as prescribed to inhibit the action of osteoclasts in bone. For hypercalcemia caused by cancer, give plicamycin (Mithracin).
- Assess the patient for arrhythmias.
- Assess for signs and symptoms of renal calculi; strain the patient's urine if needed.
- Assess for signs and symptoms of digoxin toxicity if the patient also receives digoxin (Lanoxin).

Hypocalcemia

◆ Hypocalcemia is characterized by a total serum calcium level below 8.2 mg/dl (SI, 2.05 mmol/L) and an ionized serum calcium level below 4.6 mg/dl (SI, 1.1 mmol/L).

◆ Common causes of hypocalcemia include inadequate calcium intake, calcium malabsorption, and excess calcium loss.

 AGE ALERT *Factors that contribute to hypocalcemia in geriatric patients include inadequate dietary intake of calcium, poor calcium absorption, and reduced activity or inactivity.*

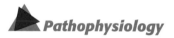 *Pathophysiology*

WHAT HAPPENS IN HYPOCALCEMIA

Calcium or vitamin D intake or absorption decreases, or calcium excretion increases.

▼

Parathyroid glands release parathyroid hormone (PTH).

▼

PTH draws calcium from bone and promotes renal reabsorption and intestinal absorption of calcium.

▼

Lack of calcium outstrips PTH's ability to compensate.

▼

Calcium is no longer available to maintain cell structure and function.

▼

Patient develops neuromuscular and cardiac symptoms and decreased level of consciousness.

Causes

◆ Inadequate calcium intake.
  – Chronic alcoholism.
  – Insufficient exposure to sunlight.
  – Possibly breast-feeding.

 AGE ALERT *A breast-fed infant can develop low calcium and vitamin D levels if the mother's intake of these nutrients is inadequate.*

◆ Calcium malabsorption.
  – Severe diarrhea.
  – Laxative abuse.
  – Malabsorption syndrome.
  – Insufficient vitamin D.
  – High phosphorus level in the intestines.
  – Reduced gastric acidity.
◆ Excess calcium loss.
  – Pancreatic insufficiency.
  – Acute pancreatitis.
  – Thyroid or parathyroid surgery.
  – Hypoparathyroidism or other parathyroid gland disorders.
  – Use of certain drugs.
◆ Other causes.
  – Severe burns and infections.
  – Hypoalbuminemia.
  – Hyperphosphatemia.
  – Alkalosis.
  – Massive blood transfusion.

DRUGS THAT CAN CAUSE HYPOCALCEMIA

◆ Anticonvulsants, especially phenytoin (Dilantin) and phenobarbital (Luminal)
◆ Calcitonin (Calcimar)
◆ Drugs that lower the serum magnesium level, such as cisplatin (Platinol-AQ) and gentamicin (Garamycin)

◆ Edetate disodium (Endrate)
◆ Loop diuretics, such as ethacrynic acid (Edecrin) and furosemide (Lasix)
◆ Plicamycin (Mithracin)
◆ Phosphates (oral, I.V., or rectal)

Signs and symptoms

- ◆ Anxiety, confusion, and irritability.
- ◆ Arrhythmias and decreased cardiac output.
- ◆ Brittle nails or dry skin and hair.
- ◆ Diarrhea.
- ◆ Diminished response to digoxin (Lanoxin).
- ◆ Hyperactive DTRs.
- ◆ Paresthesia of toes, fingers, or face, especially around the mouth.
- ◆ Spasms of laryngeal and abdominal muscles.
- ◆ Tetany, tremors, twitching, and muscle cramps.
- ◆ Trousseau's sign or Chvostek's sign.

CHECKING FOR TROUSSEAU'S AND CHVOSTEK'S SIGNS

Testing for Trousseau's and Chvostek's signs can aid in the diagnosis of tetany and hypocalcemia. Here's how to check for these important signs.

Trousseau's sign

To check for Trousseau's sign, apply a blood pressure cuff to the patient's upper arm and inflate it to a pressure 20 mm Hg above the systolic pressure. Trousseau's sign may appear after 1 to 4 minutes. The patient will experience an adducted thumb, flexed wrist and metacarpophalangeal joints, and extended interphalangeal joints (with fingers together) – carpopedal spasm – indicating tetany, a major sign of hypocalcemia.

Chvostek's sign

You can induce Chvostek's sign by tapping the patient's facial nerve adjacent to the ear. A brief contraction of the upper lip, nose, or side of the face indicates Chvostek's sign and tetany.

Diagnostic test results

- ◆ ECG changes, such as lengthened QT intervals and prolonged ST segments.
- ◆ Ionized calcium level below 4.6 mg/dl (SI, 1.1 mmol/L).
- ◆ Total serum calcium level below 8.2 mg/dl (SI, 2.05 mmol/L).

Management

♦ For a patient with acute hypocalcemia, immediately administer I.V. calcium gluconate or calcium chloride.

 ALERT *Frequently assess the I.V. site and administer I.V. calcium with an infusion pump because infiltration can cause tissue necrosis and sloughing. Never administer I.V. calcium rapidly because it may cause syncope, hypotension, and arrhythmias.*

♦ Give magnesium with calcium because hypocalcemia doesn't respond to calcium therapy alone.

♦ For a patient with chronic hypocalcemia, begin vitamin D supplementation to promote calcium absorption.

♦ Provide a diet that's rich in calcium, vitamin D, and protein.

♦ Administer a phosphate binder, such as an aluminum hydroxide antacid, to lower an elevated phosphorus level, if needed.

♦ Keep a tracheotomy tray and handheld resuscitation bag nearby in case the patient develops laryngospasm.

♦ Place the patient on a cardiac monitor to detect changes in heart rate and rhythm, especially if he's receiving digoxin (Lanoxin).

♦ Assess for Chvostek's sign and Trousseau's sign.

♦ Institute seizure precautions if indicated.

Hyperphosphatemia

◆ Hyperphosphatemia is characterized by a serum phosphorus level above 4.5 mg/dl (SI, 1.45 mmol/L).
◆ Causes of hyperphosphatemia include impaired renal excretion of phosphorus, shifting of phosphorus from intracellular to extracellular fluid, and increased dietary intake of phosphorus.

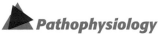 *Pathophysiology*

WHAT HAPPENS IN HYPERPHOSPHATEMIA

| Intake of phosphorus or vitamin D is excessive. | Renal insult or failure reduces glomerular filtration rate to below 30 ml/minute. |

Kidneys can't filter excess phosphorus adequately.

Phosphorus shifts from intracelluar to extracellular fluid.

Serum phosphorus level increases.

Phosphorus binds with calcium, forming insoluble compound.

Insoluable compound is deposited in lungs, heart, kidneys, eyes, skin, and other soft tissues.

Causes

◆ Impaired phosphorus excretion.
- – Hypoparathyroidism.
- – Any disorder that causes the glomerular filtration rate to fall below 30 ml/minute.
◆ Phosphorus shifting to extracellular fluid.
- – Acid-base imbalances.
- – Chemotherapy.
- – Muscle necrosis.
- – Rhabdomyolysis.
◆ Increased phosphorus intake.
- – Overuse of phosphorus supplements.
- – Overuse of phosphorus-containing laxatives or enemas.
- – Use of certain drugs.

 AGE ALERT *Infants who are fed cow's milk are predisposed to hyperphosphatemia because cow's milk contains more phosphorus than breast milk.*

DRUGS THAT CAN CAUSE HYPERPHOSPHATEMIA

◆ Enemas containing phosphorus (Fleet)
◆ Laxatives containing phosphorus or phosphate
◆ Oral phosphorus supplements (Neutra-Phos)

◆ Parenteral phosphorus supplements, such as sodium phosphate and potassium phosphate
◆ Vitamin D supplements

Signs and symptoms

◆ Anorexia, nausea, and vomiting.
◆ Arrhythmias and irregular heart rate.
◆ Chvostek's sign or Trousseau's sign.
◆ Conjunctivitis or vision impairment.
◆ Impaired mental status and seizures.
◆ Hyperreflexia.
◆ Muscle weakness, cramps, and spasms.
◆ Papular eruptions and dry, itchy skin.
◆ Paresthesia, especially in the fingertips and around the mouth.
◆ Tetany.

Diagnostic test results

◆ ECG changes, such as prolonged QT intervals and ST segments.
◆ Increased blood urea nitrogen (BUN) and creatinine levels, which reflect worsening renal function.
◆ Serum calcium level below 8.2 mg/dl (SI, 2.05 mmol/L).
◆ Serum phosphorus level above 4.5 mg/dl (SI, 1.45 mmol/L).

 ALERT *Phosphorus and calcium have an inverse relationship, meaning that hyperphosphatemia may lead to hypocalcemia, which can be life-threatening.*

◆ X-rays revealing skeletal changes caused by osteodystrophy in chronic hyperphosphatemia.

Management

- Limit the patient's phosphorus intake from dietary sources or drugs.
- Give an aluminum, magnesium, or calcium gel or phosphorus-binding antacid to decrease GI absorption of phosphorus.

     ALERT *For a patient with renal insufficiency, avoid the use of magnesium antacids because of the increased risk of hypermagnesemia.*

- Treat the underlying cause of hyperphosphatemia, such as respiratory acidosis or DKA, which can lower the serum phosphorus level.
- For a patient with severe hyperphosphatemia and normal renal function, administer I.V. saline solution to promote renal excretion of phosphorus.
- If hyperphosphatemia is related to renal failure, prepare the patient for dialysis.
- Monitor the patient for signs and symptoms of calcium phosphate calcification.
- Monitor for signs and symptoms of hypocalcemia.

SIGNS OF CALCIFICATION

Calcification usually results from chronic elevation of the serum phosphorus level. It can produce the following signs:

- arrhythmias
- conjunctivitis
- corneal haziness and impaired vision

- decreased urine output
- irregular heart rate or palpitations
- papular eruptions.

Hypophosphatemia

◆ Hypophosphatemia is characterized by a serum phosphorus level below 2.7 mg/dl (SI, 0.87 mmol/L).
◆ Generally, hypophosphatemia indicates a phosphorus deficiency. However, it can occur under circumstances when total body phosphorus stores are normal.
◆ Severe hypophosphatemia occurs when the serum phosphorus level is less then 1 mg/dl (SI, 0.3 mmol/L) and can lead to organ failure.
◆ Hypophosphatemia can result from a shifting of phosphorus from extracellular fluid to intracellular fluid, decreased intestinal absorption of phosphorus, or increased renal loss of phosphorus.

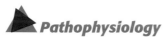 *Pathophysiology*

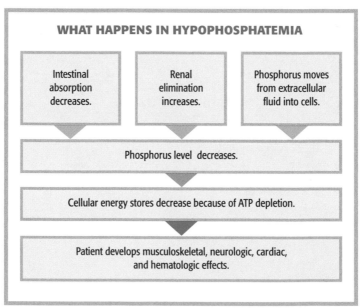

WHAT HAPPENS IN HYPOPHOSPHATEMIA

| Intestinal absorption decreases. | Renal elimination increases. | Phosphorus moves from extracellular fluid into cells. |

Phosphorus level decreases.

Cellular energy stores decrease because of ATP depletion.

Patient develops musculoskeletal, neurologic, cardiac, and hematologic effects.

Causes

◆ Phosphorus shifting to intracellular fluid.
  – Respiratory alkalosis.
  – Hyperglycemia.
  – Insulin therapy.
  – Malnourishment.
  – Hypothermia.
◆ Decreased phosphorus absorption.
  – Malabsorption syndromes.
  – Starvation.
  – Prolonged or excessive use of phosphorus-binding antacids.
  – Inadequate vitamin D intake or synthesis.
  – Diarrhea.
  – Laxative abuse.
◆ Increased renal loss of phosphorus.
  – Diuretic use.
  – DKA.
  – Alcohol abuse.
  – Hyperparathyroidism.
  – Hypocalcemia.
  – Extensive burns.

DRUGS THAT CAN CAUSE HYPOPHOSPHATEMIA

◆ Diuretics, such as acetazolamide (Diamox), loop diuretics (bumetanide [Bumex] and furosemide [Lasix]), and thiazide diuretics (chlorothiazide [Diuril] and hydrochlorothiazide [Hydro-DIURIL])
◆ Antacids, such as aluminum carbonate (Basaljel), aluminum hydroxide (Alu-Tab), calcium carbonate (Tums), and magnesium oxide (Maox 420)
◆ Insulin (Humulin, Novolin)
◆ Laxatives
◆ Phosphorus-binding drugs, such as sevelamer (Renagel) and calcium acetate (PhosLo)

Signs and symptoms

◆ Anorexia.
◆ Bruising and bleeding, particularly mild GI bleeding.
◆ Chest pain.
◆ Hypotension and low cardiac output.
◆ Irritability, apprehension, and confusion.
◆ Muscle weakness, myalgia, and malaise.
◆ Osteomalacia and bone pain.
◆ Paresthesia.
◆ Respiratory failure.
◆ Seizures and coma.

Diagnostic test results

◆ Elevated creatine kinase level, if rhabdomyolysis is present.
◆ Serum phosphorus level below 2.7 mg/dl (SI, 0.87 mmol/L).
◆ X-rays revealing skeletal changes caused by osteomalacia or bone fractures.

Management

◆ If hypophosphatemia is mild, encourage the patient to eat a high-phosphorus diet.

◆ If the patient has moderate hypophosphatemia or can't consume phosphorus-rich foods, provide oral supplements.

◆ If hypophosphatemia is severe, replace the deficient electrolyte with I.V. potassium phosphate or sodium phosphate.

 ALERT *Administer potassium phosphate slowly (no faster than 10 mEq/hour [SI, 10 mmol/hr]). Adverse effects of too-rapid I.V. replacement for hypophosphatemia include hyperphosphatemia and hypocalcemia.*

◆ Assess the patient's medication history.

 AGE ALERT *A geriatric patient's drugs can alter electrolyte levels by affecting phosphorus absorption. Be sure to ask if the patient uses over-the-counter drugs, such as antacids or laxatives.*

◆ Monitor for "refeeding syndrome" when a patient starts TPN therapy. This syndrome, which causes phosphorus to shift into cells, usually occurs 3 or more days after TPN begins.

◆ Closely monitor the results of arterial blood gas (ABG) analysis and pulse oximetry to detect respiratory changes.

◆ Closely monitor the patient's cardiac and neurologic status.

◆ Take seizure precautions if needed.

Hyperchloremia

◆ Hyperchloremia is characterized by a serum chloride level above 106 mEq/L (SI, 106 mmol/L).

 AGE ALERT *In patients between ages 60 and 90, the normal serum chloride level ranges from 98 to 107 mEq/L (SI, 98 to 107 mmol/L); in patients age 90 and older, from 98 to 111 mEq/L (SI, 98 to 111 mmol/L).*

◆ In hyperchloremia, excess chloride in extracellular fluid is linked to other electrolyte imbalances. Therefore, it rarely occurs alone.

◆ Causes of hyperchloremia include increased chloride intake or absorption, acidosis, and chloride retention by the kidneys.

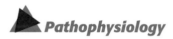 *Pathophysiology*

WHAT HAPPENS IN HYPERCHLOREMIA

Chloride intake, absorption, or retention increases.

Water loss may worsen chloride accumulation in extracellular fluid.

Bicarbonate level falls, and sodium level rises.

Patient develops signs and symptoms of metabolic acidosis.

Causes

- Increased chloride intake or absorption.
  - Overconsumption of sodium chloride.
  - Water loss.
  - Anastomoses of the ureter and intestines.
- Acidosis.
  - Dehydration.
  - Renal tubular acidosis.
  - Renal failure.
  - Respiratory alkalosis.
  - Salicylate toxicity.
  - Hyperparathyroidism.
  - Hyperaldosteronism.
  - Hypernatremia.
- Chloride retention by the kidneys.
  - Use of certain drugs.

DRUGS THAT CAN CAUSE HYPERCHLOREMIA

- Acetazolamide (Diamox)
- Ammonium chloride
- Phenylbutazone (Butazolidin)
- Salicylates such as aspirin (Bufferin), with overdose
- Sodium polystyrene sulfonate (Kayexalate)
- Triamterene (Dyrenium)

Signs and symptoms

◆ Arrhythmias and decreased cardiac output.
◆ Decreased LOC, possibly progressing to coma.
◆ Dyspnea.
◆ Fluid retention and edema.
◆ Kussmaul's respirations.
◆ Lethargy.
◆ Other signs and symptoms of metabolic acidosis.
◆ Tachycardia and hypertension.
◆ Tachypnea.
◆ Weakness.

Diagnostic test results

◆ Serum chloride level above 106 mEq/L (SI, 106 mmol/L).
◆ Serum pH below 7.35 (SI, 7.35), serum bicarbonate level below 22 mEq/L (SI, 22 mmol/L), and normal anion gap (8 to 14 mEq/L [SI, 8 to 14 mmol/L]), suggesting metabolic acidosis.
◆ Serum sodium level above 145 mEq/L (SI, 145 mmol/L).

Management

♦ Focus on restoring the patient's fluid, electrolyte, and acid-base balance.

♦ Restrict the patient's sodium and chloride intake.

♦ Administer a diuretic to promote chloride elimination, if the patient isn't dehydrated.

♦ For a dehydrated patient, administer fluids to dilute the blood and force renal excretion of chloride.

♦ In a patient with adequate liver function, correct acidosis by infusing lactated Ringer's solution as prescribed.

♦ If hyperchloremia is severe, administer I.V. sodium bicarbonate to raise the serum bicarbonate level.

♦ Closely monitor the patient's cardiac rhythm to detect changes.

♦ If the patient is receiving I.V. bicarbonate, monitor for signs and symptoms of metabolic alkalosis, which may result from over-correction.

Hypochloremia

- ◆ Hypochloremia is characterized by a serum chloride level below 96 mEq/L (SI, 96 mmol/L).
- ◆ In hypochloremia, a chloride deficiency exists in extracellular fluid.
- ◆ A decrease in the serum chloride level can affect the levels of sodium, potassium, calcium, and other electrolytes.
- ◆ Causes of hypochloremia include decreased chloride intake, increased chloride loss, and sodium or acid-base imbalances.

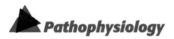

Pathophysiology

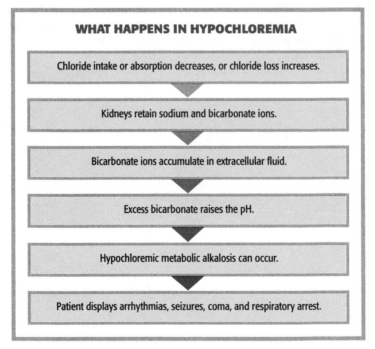

WHAT HAPPENS IN HYPOCHLOREMIA

Chloride intake or absorption decreases, or chloride loss increases.

Kidneys retain sodium and bicarbonate ions.

Bicarbonate ions accumulate in extracellular fluid.

Excess bicarbonate raises the pH.

Hypochloremic metabolic alkalosis can occur.

Patient displays arrhythmias, seizures, coma, and respiratory arrest.

Causes

- Decreased chloride intake.
  - Use of chloride-deficient formula in infants.
  - Salt-restricted diet.
  - Therapy with I.V. fluids that lack chloride.
- Increased chloride loss.
  - Prolonged vomiting.
  - Diarrhea.
  - Severe diaphoresis.
  - Gastric surgery.
  - NG tube suctioning.
  - Other GI tube drainage.
  - Cystic fibrosis.
  - Use of certain drugs.
- Other imbalances.
  - Sodium deficiency.
  - Potassium deficiency.
  - Metabolic alkalosis.
  - Conditions that affect acid-base or electrolyte balance, such as DKA, Addison's disease, and heart failure.

DRUGS THAT CAN CAUSE HYPOCHLOREMIA

- Loop diuretics such as furosemide (Lasix)
- Osmotic diuretics such as mannitol (Osmitrol)
- Thiazide diuretics such as hydrochlorothiazide (HydroDIURIL)

Signs and symptoms

- ◆ Agitation and irritability.
- ◆ Arrhythmias.
- ◆ Hyperactive DTRs.
- ◆ Muscle cramps and weakness.
- ◆ Muscle hypertonicity.
- ◆ Seizures or coma.
- ◆ Slow, shallow respirations or respiratory arrest.
- ◆ Other signs and symptoms of metabolic alkalosis.
- ◆ Tetany.
- ◆ Twitching.

Diagnostic test results

- ◆ Serum chloride level below 96 mEq/L (96 mmol/L).
- ◆ Serum pH above 7.45 (SI, 7.45) and serum bicarbonate level above 26 mEq/L (SI, 26 mmol/L), suggesting metabolic alkalosis.
- ◆ Serum sodium level below 135 mEq/L (SI 135 mmol/L), indicating hyponatremia.

Management

◆ Replace chloride by administering I.V. fluids, such as normal saline solution, or drugs and encouraging increased dietary intake of chloride.

◆ Treat accompanying metabolic alkalosis or electrolyte imbalances as indicated.

◆ Treat the underlying cause of renal or GI loss of chloride, for example, by withholding a diuretic or giving an antiemetic.

◆ Monitor the patient's LOC, muscle strength, and movement.

◆ Observe for worsening respiratory function. Keep emergency equipment nearby.

◆ Monitor the patient's cardiac rhythm.

◆ If administering ammonium chloride to correct metabolic acidosis, assess the patient for pain at the infusion site and adjust the rate if needed.

 ALERT *Don't give ammonium chloride to a patient with severe hepatic disease because the drug is metabolized by the liver.*

◆ Use normal saline solution — not tap water — to flush the patient's NG tube.

4

Acid-base imbalances

Respiratory acidosis

◆ A compromise in any essential part of breathing — ventilation, perfusion, or diffusion — may lead to respiratory acidosis.

◆ In respiratory acidosis, the pulmonary system can't rid the body of enough carbon dioxide (CO_2) to maintain a healthy pH (hydrogen ion) balance.

◆ Respiratory acidosis may be acute, in which the pH falls abnormally low (below 7.35 [SI, 7.35]).

◆ Respiratory acidosis may be chronic, in which the pH stays within normal limits (7.34 to 7.45 [SI, 7.34 to 7.45]) because the kidneys have time to compensate for the imbalance.

◆ This imbalance can result from neuromuscular problems, depression of the respiratory center in the brain, lung diseases, or an airway obstruction.

 Pathophysiology

WHAT HAPPENS IN RESPIRATORY ACIDOSIS

This series of illustrations shows at the cellular level how respiratory acidosis develops.

Step 1

When pulmonary ventilation decreases, retained carbon dioxide (CO_2) combines with water to form carbonic acid (H_2CO_3) in

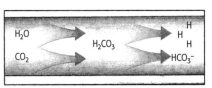

larger than normal amounts. The carbonic acid dissociates to release free hydrogen ions (H) and bicarbonate ions (HCO_3^-). The excess carbonic acid causes a drop in pH. *Look for a Paco$_2$ level above 45 mm Hg (SI, 5.3 kPa) and a pH level below 7.35 (SI, 7.35).*

Step 2

As the pH level falls, 2,3-diphosphoglycerate (2,3-DPG) increases in the red blood cells and causes a change in hemoglobin (Hb) that makes the hemoglobin release oxygen

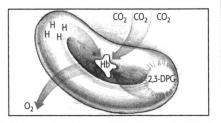

WHAT HAPPENS IN RESPIRATORY ACIDOSIS *(continued)*

(O_2). The altered hemoglobin, now strongly alkaline, picks up hydrogen ions and CO_2, thus eliminating some of the free hydrogen ions and excess CO_2. *Look for decreased arterial oxygen saturation.*

Step 3

Whenever $Paco_2$ increases, CO_2 builds up in all tissues and fluids, including cerebrospinal fluid and the respiratory center in the medulla. The CO_2 reacts with water to form carbonic acid, which then breaks into free hydrogen ions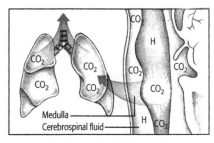
and bicarbonate ions. The increased amount of CO_2 and free hydrogen ions stimulate the respiratory center to increase the respiratory rate. An increased respiratory rate expels more CO_2 and helps to reduce the CO_2 level in the blood and other tissues. *Look for rapid, shallow respirations and a decreasing $Paco_2$.*

Step 4

Eventually, CO_2 and hydrogen ions cause cerebral blood vessels to dilate, which increases blood flow to brain. That increased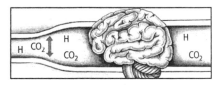
flow can cause cerebral edema and depress central nervous system activity. *Look for headache, confusion, lethargy, nausea, or vomiting.*

Step 5

As respiratory mechanisms fail, the increasing $Paco_2$ stimulates the kidneys to conserve bicarbonate and sodium ions and to excrete hydrogen ions, some in the form of ammonium (NH_4). The additional bicarbonate and sodium combine to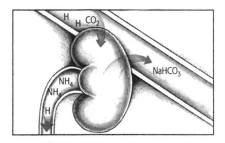
form extra sodium bicarbonate ($NaHCO_3$), which is then able to buffer more free hydrogen ions. *Look for increased acid content in the urine, increasing serum pH and bicarbonate levels, and shallow, depressed respirations.*

(continued)

WHAT HAPPENS IN RESPIRATORY ACIDOSIS *(continued)*

Step 6

As the concentration of hydrogen ions overwhelms the body's compensatory mechanisms, the hydrogen ions move into the cells, and potassium ions (K) move out. A concurrent lack of oxygen causes an increase in the anaerobic production of lactic acid, which further skews the acid-base balance and critically depresses neurologic and cardiac functions. *Look for hyperkalemia, arrhythmias, increased $Paco_2$, decreased pH, and decreased level of consciousness.*

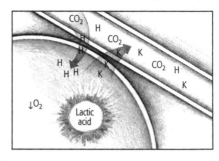

Causes

- ◆ Neuromuscular problems.
  - – Guillain-Barré syndrome.
  - – Myasthenia gravis.
  - – Poliomyelitis.
  - – Spinal cord injury.
- ◆ Respiratory center depression.
  - – Central nervous system (CNS) trauma.
  - – Brain lesions.
  - – Obesity.
  - – Primary hypoventilation.
  - – Use of certain drugs.
- ◆ Lung diseases.
  - – Respiratory infections.
  - – Chronic obstructive pulmonary disease (COPD).
  - – Acute asthma attacks.
  - – Chronic bronchitis.
  - – Acute respiratory distress syndrome.
  - – Pulmonary edema.
  - – Chest wall trauma.
- ◆ Airway obstruction.
  - – Retained secretions.
  - – Tumors.
  - – Anaphylaxis.
  - – Laryngeal spasm.
  - – Lung diseases that alter alveolar ventilation.

 AGE ALERT *Children are especially prone to airway obstruction. So are geriatric and debilitated patients, who may not be able to effectively clear secretions.*

Infants commonly have problems with acid-base imbalances, particularly acidosis. Their low residual lung volume allows any change in respirations to alter their partial pressure of arterial carbon dioxide ($PaCO_2$), leading to acidosis. Their high metabolic rate yields large amounts of metabolic wastes and acids that must be excreted by the kidneys. Together with their immature buffer system, this leaves infants prone to acidosis.

DRUGS THAT CAN CAUSE RESPIRATORY ACIDOSIS

Anesthetics
- enflurane (Ethrane)
- halothane (Fluothane)
- isoflurane (Forane)
- nitrous oxide

Opioids
- butorphanol (Stadol)
- meperidine (Demerol)
- morphine (Duramorph)
- nalbuphine (Nubain)

Sedatives and hypnotics
- amobarbital (Amytal)
- chloral hydrate (Noctec)
- estazolam (ProSom)
- flurazepam (Dalmane)
- lorazepam (Ativan)
- pentobarbital (Nembutal)
- secobarbital (Seconal)
- triazolam (Halcion)

Signs and symptoms

- Tachycardia.
- Dyspnea with rapid, shallow respirations.
- Nausea and vomiting.
- Decreased deep tendon reflexes.
- Warm, flushed skin.
- Diaphoresis.
- Restlessness.
- Tremors.
- Apprehension.
- Confusion and decreasing level of consciousness (LOC).

Diagnostic test results

◆ Arterial blood gas (ABG) analysis.

ABG RESULTS IN RESPIRATORY ACIDOSIS

This chart shows typical arterial blood gas (ABG) levels in uncompensated and compensated respiratory acidosis.

ABG	Uncompensated	Compensated
pH	< 7.35 (SI, < 7.35)	Normal
$Paco_2$	> 45 mm Hg (SI, > 5.3 kPa)	> 45 mm Hg (SI, > 5.3 kPa)
HCO_3^-	Normal	> 26 mEq/L (SI, > 26 mmol/L)

◆ Chest X-rays.
  – Evidence of COPD.
  – Evidence of pneumonia, pneumothorax, or other cause.
◆ Electrolyte levels.
  – Potassium level above 5 mEq/L (SI, 5 mmol/L).
◆ Other blood tests.
  – Drug screening that may detect overdose.

Management

◆ Maintain a patent airway.
◆ Give a bronchodilator to open constricted airways.
◆ Administer supplemental oxygen as needed.

 ALERT *Expect to use a lower oxygen concentration for a patient with COPD. In such a patient, the medulla is accustomed to high CO_2 levels, and a lack of oxygen stimulates breathing. Therefore, administration of too much oxygen can diminish the stimulus to breathe and depress respiratory efforts.*

◆ Give drugs to treat hyperkalemia.
◆ Give an antibiotic to treat infection.
◆ Perform chest physiotherapy to remove secretions from the lungs.
◆ Perform tracheal suctioning, incentive spirometry, and postural drainage, and assist with coughing and deep breathing as needed.
◆ Monitor for changes in the patient's cardiac rhythm and respiratory pattern.
◆ Closely observe the patient's neurologic status and report significant changes.
◆ Promote fluid intake and carefully track fluid intake and output.

Respiratory alkalosis

- ◆ Respiratory alkalosis results from alveolar hyperventilation and hypocapnia.
- ◆ In respiratory alkalosis, the pH exceeds 7.45 (SI, 7.45), and the $Paco_2$ is below 35 mm Hg (SI, 4.7 kPa).
- ◆ Alkalosis may be acute, resulting from a sudden increase in ventilation, or chronic, which may be difficult to identify because of renal compensation.
- ◆ Any condition that increases the respiratory rate or depth can cause the lungs to eliminate too much CO_2. Because CO_2 is an acid, eliminating it decreases the $Paco_2$ and increases the pH.

 Pathophysiology

WHAT HAPPENS IN RESPIRATORY ALKALOSIS

This series of illustrations shows at the cellular level how respiratory alkalosis develops.

Step 1

When pulmonary ventilation increases above the amount needed to maintain normal carbon dioxide (CO_2) levels, excessive amounts of CO_2 are exhaled. This causes hypocapnia (a fall in $Paco_2$),

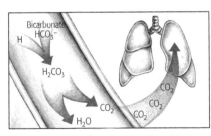

which leads to a reduction in carbonic acid (H_2CO_3) production, a loss of hydrogen ions (H) and bicarbonate ions (HCO_3^-), and a subsequent rise in pH. *Look for a pH level above 7.45 (SI, 7.45), a $Paco_2$ level below 35 mm Hg (SI, 4.7 kPa), and a bicarbonate level below 22 mEq/L (SI, 22 mmol/L).*

Step 2

In defense against the rising pH, hydrogen ions are pulled out of the cells and into the blood in exchange for potassium ions (K). The hydrogen ions entering the blood combine with bicar-

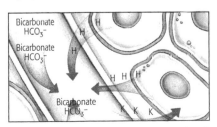

(continued)

WHAT HAPPENS IN RESPIRATORY ALKALOSIS (continued)

bonate ions to form carbonic acid, which lowers the pH. *Look for a further decrease in bicarbonate levels, a fall in pH, and a fall in serum potassium levels (hypokalemia).*

Step 3

Hypocapnia stimulates the carotid and aortic bodies and the medulla, which causes an increase in heart rate without an increase in blood pressure. *Look for angina, electrocardiogram changes, restlessness, and anxiety.*

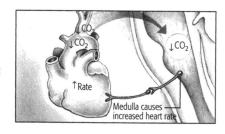

Step 4

Simultaneously, hypocapnia produces cerebral vasoconstriction, which prompts a reduction in cerebral blood flow. Hypocapnia also overexcites the medulla, pons, and other parts of the

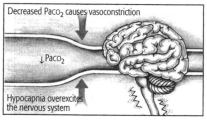

autonomic nervous system. *Look for increasing anxiety, diaphoresis, dyspnea, alternating periods of apnea and hyperventilation, dizziness, and tingling in the fingers or toes.*

Step 5

When hypocapnia lasts more than 6 hours, the kidneys increase secretion of bicarbonate and reduce excretion of hydrogen. Periods of apnea may result if the pH remains high and the $Paco_2$

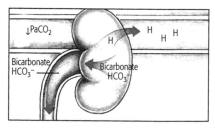

remains low. *Look for slowing of the respiratory rate, hypoventilation, and Cheyne-Stokes respirations.*

WHAT HAPPENS IN RESPIRATORY ALKALOSIS *(continued)*

Step 6

Continued low $Paco_2$ increases cerebral and peripheral hypoxia from vasoconstriction. Severe alkalosis inhibits calcium (Ca) ionization, which in turn causes increased nerve excitability and muscle contractions. Eventually, the

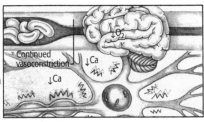

alkalosis overwhelms the central nervous system and the heart. *Look for decreasing level of consciousness, hyperreflexia, carpopedal spasm, tetany, arrhythmias, seizures, and coma.*

Causes

- ◆ Hyperventilation.
  - – Pain.
  - – Anxiety.
  - – Salicylate intoxication.
  - – Use of certain drugs.
- ◆ Hypermetabolic states.
  - – Fever.
  - – Liver failure.
  - – Sepsis.
- ◆ Conditions that affect the respiratory control center.
- ◆ Other causes.
  - – Acute hypoxia secondary to high altitude.
  - – Pulmonary disease.
  - – Severe anemia.
  - – Pulmonary embolus.
  - – Hypotension.

DRUGS THAT CAN CAUSE RESPIRATORY ALKALOSIS

Catecholamines
- ◆ dobutamine (Dobutrex)
- ◆ dopamine (Intropin)
- ◆ epinephrine (Bronkaid Mist)
- ◆ isoproterenol (Isuprel)
- ◆ norepinephrine (Levophed)

Salicylates
- ◆ aspirin (Ascriptin)
- ◆ aspirin-containing compounds
- ◆ diflunisal (Dolobid)

Xanthines
- ◆ aminophylline (Truphylline)
- ◆ oxtriphylline (Choledyl SA)
- ◆ theophylline (Theobid)

Other
- ◆ nicotine (Nicotrol)

Signs and symptoms

◆ Tachycardia.
◆ Syncope.
◆ Dyspnea and increased respiratory rate and depth.
◆ Diaphoresis.
◆ Hyperreflexia.
◆ Paresthesia.
◆ Tetany.
◆ Anxiety.
◆ Confusion.
◆ Restlessness.

Diagnostic test results

◆ ABG analysis.

ABG RESULTS IN RESPIRATORY ALKALOSIS

This chart shows typical arterial blood gas (ABG) levels in uncompensated and compensated respiratory alkalosis.

ABG	Uncompensated	Compensated
pH	> 7.45 (SI, > 7.45)	Normal
$Paco_2$	< 35 mm Hg (SI, < 4.7 kPa)	< 35 mm Hg (SI, < 4.7 kPa)
HCO_3^-	Normal	< 22 mEq/L (SI, < 22 mmol/L)

◆ Electrocardiogram (ECG) changes.
  – Arrhythmias.
  – Characteristic indications of hypokalemia or hypocalcemia.
◆ Electrolyte levels.
  – Serum calcium level below normal.
  – Serum potassium level below normal.
◆ Other blood tests.
  – Toxicology screening with evidence of salicylate poisoning.

Management

- Correct the underlying cause, for example, by treating salicylate intoxication or sepsis.
- Administer supplemental oxygen if needed.
- Give a sedative if anxiety is the cause.
- Counteract hyperventilation by instructing the patient to breath into a paper bag, which forces him to breathe exhaled CO_2 and raises the CO_2 level.
- If the cause is iatrogenic, adjust the ventilator settings.
- Monitor vital signs. Report changes in neurologic, neuromuscular, or cardiovascular functioning.
- Monitor ABG and serum electrolyte levels, and immediately report any changes.
- Take seizure precautions as needed.

Metabolic acidosis

- Metabolic acidosis is characterized by a pH below 7.35 (SI, 7.35) and a bicarbonate level below 22 mEq/L (SI, 22 mmol/L).
- This imbalance depresses the CNS and, if untreated, can lead to arrhythmias, coma, and cardiac arrest.
- Generally, metabolic acidosis is caused by bicarbonate loss from extracellular fluid, metabolic acid accumulation, or both.
- This imbalance can result from ketone overproduction, lactic acidosis, kidney disorders, GI disorders, and the use of certain drugs.

 Pathophysiology

WHAT HAPPENS IN METABOLIC ACIDOSIS

This series of illustrations shows at the cellular level how metabolic acidosis develops.

Step 1

As hydrogen ions (H) start to accumulate in the body, chemical buffers (plasma bicarbonate and proteins) in the cells and extracellular fluid bind with them. *No signs are detectable at this stage.*

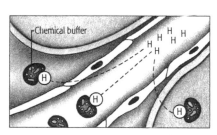

Step 2

Excess hydrogen ions that the buffers can't bind with decrease the pH and stimulate chemoreceptors in the medulla to increase the respiratory rate. The increased respiratory rate lowers the $Paco_2$, which

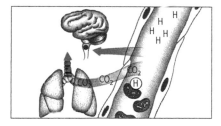

allows more hydrogen ions to bind with bicarbonate ions (HCO_3^-). Respiratory compensation occurs within minutes but isn't sufficient to correct the imbalance. *Look for a pH level below 7.35 (SI, 7.35), a bicarbonate level below 22 mEq/L (SI, 22 mmol/L), a decreasing $Paco_2$ level, and rapid, deeper respirations.*

(continued)

WHAT HAPPENS IN METABOLIC ACIDOSIS *(continued)*

Step 3

Healthy kidneys try to compensate for acidosis by secreting excess hydrogen ions into the renal tubules. Those ions are buffered by phosphate or ammonia and then are excreted into the urine in the form of a weak acid. *Look for acidic urine.*

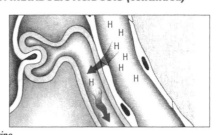

Step 4

Each time a hydrogen ion is secreted into the renal tubules, a sodium ion (Na) and a bicarbonate ion are absorbed from the tubules and returned to the blood. *Look for pH and bicarbonate levels that return slowly to normal.*

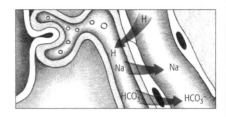

Step 5

Excess hydrogen ions in the extracellular fluid diffuse into cells. To maintain the balance of the charge across the membrane, the cells release potassium ions (K) into the blood. *Look for signs and symptoms of hyperkalemia,*

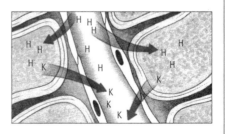

including colic and diarrhea, weakness or flaccid paralysis, tingling and numbness in the extremities, bradycardia, a tall T wave, a prolonged PR interval, and a wide QRS complex.

Step 6

Excess hydrogen ions alter the normal balance of potassium, sodium, and calcium ions (Ca), leading to reduced excitability of nerve cells. *Look for signs and symptoms of progressive central nervous system depression, including lethargy, dull headache, confusion, stupor, and coma.*

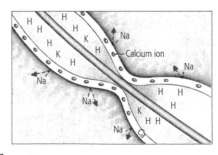

Causes

- Ketone overproduction.
  - Diabetes mellitus.
  - Chronic alcoholism.
  - Severe malnutrition.
  - Starvation.
  - Hyperthyroidism.
  - Severe infection with fever.
- Lactic acidosis.
  - Shock.
  - Heart failure.
  - Pulmonary disease.
  - Hepatic disorders.
  - Seizures.
  - Strenuous exercise.
- Kidney disorders.
  - Renal insufficiency.
  - Renal failure with acute tubular necrosis.
- GI disorders.
  - Diarrhea.
  - Intestinal malabsorption.
  - Pancreatic or hepatic fistula.
  - Urinary diversion to the ileum.
  - Hyperaldosteronism.

DRUGS THAT CAN CAUSE METABOLIC ACIDOSIS

Potassium-sparing diuretics
- acetazolamide (Diamox)
- amiloride (Midamor)
- spironolactone (Aldactone)
- triamterene (Dyrenium)

Other drugs and substances (with poisoning or toxicity)
- ammonium chloride
- aspirin or other salicylates
- ethylene glycol
- hydrochloric acid
- methanol

Signs and symptoms

◆ Hyperkalemic signs and symptoms.
  – Abdominal cramps.
  – Diarrhea.
  – Muscle weakness.
◆ Weakness.
◆ Decreased deep tendon reflexes.
◆ Hypotension.
◆ Warm, dry skin.
◆ Lethargy.
◆ Anorexia, nausea, and vomiting.
◆ Confusion and decreasing LOC.
◆ Dull headache.
◆ Kussmaul's (rapid, deep) respirations.

Diagnostic test results

◆ ABG analysis.

ABG RESULTS IN METABOLIC ACIDOSIS

This chart shows typical arterial blood gas (ABG) levels in uncompensated and compensated metabolic acidosis.

ABG	Uncompensated	Compensated
pH	< 7.35 (SI, < 7.35)	Normal
Paco$_2$	Normal	< 35 mm Hg (SI, < 4.7 kPa)
HCO$_3^-$	< 22 mEq/L (SI, < 22 mmol/L)	< 22 mEq/L (SI, < 22 mmol/L)

◆ ECG changes characteristic of hyperkalemia.
  – Tall T waves.
  – Prolonged PR intervals.
  – Wide QRS complexes.
◆ Electrolyte levels.
  – Serum potassium level above normal.
  – Increased anion gap (difference between the amount of sodium and bicarbonate in the blood).
  – Plasma lactate level above normal in patients with lactic acidosis.
◆ Other blood tests.
  – Blood glucose and serum ketone levels above normal in patients with diabetic ketoacidosis (DKA).

Management

◆ Promote respiratory compensation, for example, by providing mechanical ventilation.
◆ Administer a rapid-acting insulin to reverse DKA and move potassium back into cells.
◆ Monitor the patient's potassium level.
◆ Administer sodium bicarbonate I.V. to neutralize blood acidity if the patient's pH is less than 7.1 (SI, 7.1).

 ALERT *Flush the I.V. line with normal saline solution before and after administering sodium bicarbonate because the bicarbonate may inactivate or cause precipitation of other drugs. Be aware that too much bicarbonate can cause metabolic alkalosis and pulmonary edema.*

◆ Begin dialysis for a patient with renal failure or a toxic drug reaction.

 ALERT *If dopamine doesn't raise the blood pressure, check the patient's blood pH. A pH below 7.1 (SI, 7.1) causes resistance to vasopressors such as dopamine. To make dopamine more effective, correct the patient's pH.*

◆ Give an antidiarrheal if the bicarbonate loss has been caused by diarrhea.
◆ Closely monitor the patient's neurologic status to detect changes in LOC and CNS deterioration.

Metabolic alkalosis

◆ Metabolic alkalosis is characterized by a blood pH above 7.45 (SI, 7.45) and a bicarbonate level above 26 mEq/L (SI, 26 mmol/L).

◆ If untreated, this condition can lead to coma, arrhythmias, and death.

◆ Generally, metabolic alkalosis results from a loss of hydrogen ions (acid), a gain of bicarbonate ions, or both.

 Pathophysiology

WHAT HAPPENS IN METABOLIC ALKALOSIS

This series of illustrations shows at the cellular level how metabolic alkalosis develops.

Step 1

As bicarbonate ions (HCO_3^-) start to accumulate in the body, chemical buffers (in extracellular fluid and cells) bind with the ions. *No signs are detectable at this stage.*

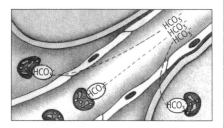

Step 2

Excess bicarbonate ions that don't bind with chemical buffers elevate serum pH levels, which in turn depress chemoreceptors in the medulla. Depression of those chemoreceptors causes a decrease in respiratory rate, which increases

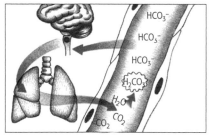

the $Paco_2$. The additional carbon dioxide (CO_2) combines with water to form carbonic acid (H_2CO_3). Note: Lowered oxygen levels limit respiratory compensation. *Look for a serum pH level above 7.45 (SI, 7.45), a bicarbonate level above 26 mEq/L (SI, 26 mmol/L), a rising $Paco_2$, and slow shallow respirations.*

(continued)

WHAT HAPPENS IN METABOLIC ALKALOSIS *(continued)*

Step 3

When the bicarbonate level exceeds 28 mEq/L (SI, 28 mmol/L), the renal glomeruli can no longer reabsorb excess bicarbonate. That excess bicarbonate is excreted in the urine; hydrogen ions are retained. *Look for alkaline urine and pH and bicarbonate levels that return slowly to normal.*

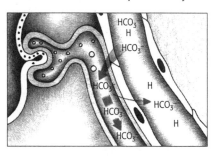

Step 4

To maintain electrochemical balance, the kidneys excrete excess sodium ions (Na), water, and bicarbonate. *Look for polyuria initially, then signs and symptoms of hypovolemia, including thirst and dry mucous membranes.*

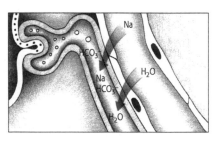

Step 5

Lowered hydrogen ion levels in the extracellular fluid cause the ions to diffuse out of the cells. To maintain the balance of charge across the cell membrane, extracellular potassium ions (K) move into the cells. *Look for signs and symptoms of hypokalemia, including anorexia, muscle weakness, loss of reflexes, and others.*

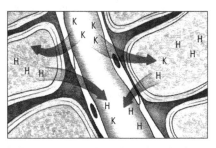

WHAT HAPPENS IN METABOLIC ALKALOSIS *(continued)*

Step 6

As hydrogen ion levels decline, calcium (Ca) ionization decreases. That decrease in ionization makes nerve cells more permeable to sodium ions. Sodium ions moving into nerve cells stimulate neural impulses and produce overexcitability of the peripheral and central nervous systems. *Look for tetany, belligerance, irritability, disorientation, and seizures.*

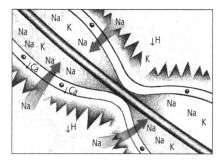

Causes

- Hypokalema.
  - Use of diuretics.
  - Use of other drugs.
- Excessive acid loss from the GI tract.
  - Vomiting.
  - Pyloric stenosis.
  - Nasogastric (NG) suctioning.
- Other causes.
  - Cushing's disease.
  - Overcorrection of acidosis.
  - Kidney disease such as renal artery stenosis.
  - Multiple transfusions.

DRUGS THAT CAN CAUSE METABOLIC ALKALOSIS

Antacids
- calcium carbonate (Tums)
- sodium bicarbonate (Bell/ans)

Loop diuretics
- bumetanide (Bumex)
- ethacrynic acid (Edecrin)
- furosemide (Lasix)

Thiazide diuretics
- chlorothiazide (Diuril)
- hydrochlorothiazide (Hydro-DIURIL)

Signs and symptoms

- ◆ Hypotension.
- ◆ Cyanosis.
- ◆ Nausea and vomiting.
- ◆ Anorexia.
- ◆ Weakness.
- ◆ Paresthesia.
- ◆ Hyperactive reflexes.
- ◆ Muscle twitching and tetany.
- ◆ Polyuria.
- ◆ Apathy and confusion.

Diagnostic test results

- ◆ ABG analysis.

ABG RESULTS IN METABOLIC ALKALOSIS

This chart shows typical arterial blood gas (ABG) levels in uncompensated and compensated metabolic alkalosis.

ABG	Uncompensated	Compensated
pH	> 7.45 (SI, > 7.45)	Normal
$Paco_2$	Normal	> 45 mm Hg (SI, > 5.3 kPa)
HCO_3^-	> 26 mEq/L (SI, > 26 mmol/L)	> 26 mEq/L (SI, > 26 mmol/L)

- ◆ ECG.
  - – Low T waves that merge with P waves.
- ◆ Electrolyte levels.
  - – Serum potassium, calcium, and chloride levels below normal.

Management

◆ For severe metabolic alkalosis, administer ammonium chloride I.V.

 ALERT *Infuse 0.9% ammonium chloride no faster than 1 L over 4 hours. Faster administration can cause hemolysis of red blood cells. Don't give this drug to a patient with hepatic or renal disease.*

◆ Discontinue thiazide diuretics and NG suctioning.
◆ Give an antiemetic to treat underlying nausea and vomiting.
◆ Give acetazolamide (Diamox) to increase renal excretion of bicarbonate.
◆ Administer supplemental oxygen as needed, to correct hypoxemia.
◆ Take seizure precautions as needed.
◆ Administer a diluted potassium solution, using an infusion pump.
◆ Irrigate an NG tube with normal saline solution instead of tap water, to prevent the loss of gastric electrolytes.
◆ Monitor the patient closely for muscle weakness, tetany, or decreased muscular activity.

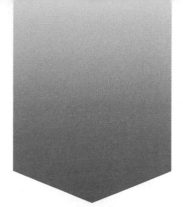

5

Disorders that cause imbalances

Heart failure

◆ Heart failure is a syndrome of myocardial dysfunction that causes diminished cardiac output.

◆ Heart failure occurs when the heart can't pump enough blood to meet the body's metabolic needs.

◆ Any alteration in preload (volume), afterload (pressure), contractility (squeeze), or heart rate can decrease cardiac output and lead to heart failure.

◆ Normally, the pumping actions of the right and left sides of the heart complement each other, producing a synchronized and continuous blood flow.

◆ When a disorder occurs, one side of the heart may fail while the other continues to function normally for a time.

◆ If one side of the heart fails, the resulting strain eventually causes the other side to fail, resulting in total heart failure.

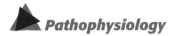

Pathophysiology

WHAT HAPPENS IN HEART FAILURE

Left-sided heart failure	Right-sided heart failure

Left ventricular contractility diminishes.

Right ventricular contractility diminishes.

Left ventricle's ability to pump fails, producing increased heart rate, pale cool skin, arm and leg tingling, and arrhythmias.

Right ventricle's ability to pump fails, producing increased heart rate, cool skin, cyanosis, and arrhythmias.

Cardiac output to the body decreases.

Cardiac output to the lungs decreases.

Blood backs up into left atrium and lungs, causing dyspnea on exertion, confusion, dizziness, orthostatic hypotension, decreased peripheral pulses and pulse pressure, cyanosis, and S_3 gallop.

Blood backs up into right atrium and peripheral circulation, causing weight gain, peripheral edema, and engorgement of kidneys and other organs.

Pulmonary congestion, dyspnea, and activity intolerance occur.

Pulmonary edema occurs.

Patient may develop right-sided failure if right ventricle becomes stressed from pumping against greater pulmonary resistance.

Causes

- ◆ Myocardial infarction.
- ◆ Myocardial fibrosis.
- ◆ Ventricular overload.
- ◆ Restricted ventricular diastolic filling.

Imbalances caused by heart failure

- ◆ Hypervolemia and hypovolemia.
- ◆ Hyperkalemia and hypokalemia.
- ◆ Hypochloremia.
- ◆ Hypomagnesemia.
- ◆ Hyponatremia.
- ◆ Metabolic acidosis and alkalosis.
- ◆ Respiratory acidosis and alkalosis.

Signs and symptoms

Left-sided heart failure

◆ Third and fourth heart sounds.
◆ Tachycardia.
◆ Exertional dyspnea and paroxysmal nocturnal dyspnea.
◆ Orthopnea and tachypnea.
◆ Coughing, possibly with pink, frothy sputum.
◆ Wheezes and crackles.
◆ Oliguria.
◆ Decreasing level of consciousness.
◆ Fatigue.
◆ Weakness.

Right-sided heart failure

◆ Arrhythmias.
◆ Chest tightness.
◆ Neck vein distention and rigidity.
◆ Venous engorgement.
◆ Palpitations.
◆ Peripheral edema and ascites.
◆ Cyanotic nail beds.
◆ Anorexia and nausea.
◆ Cool, clammy skin.
◆ Cardiac arrest.

Diagnostic test results

◆ Chest X-rays.
  – Edema.
  – Effusion.
  – Congestion.
◆ Echocardiograms.
  – Enlarged heart chambers.
  – Changes in ventricular function.
◆ Electrocardiogram (ECG) tracings.
  – Arrhythmias.
◆ Hemodynamic pressure readings.
  – Increased central venous pressure.
  – Increased pulmonary artery wedge pressure.

Management

♦ Place the patient in Fowler's position, and administer supplemental oxygen to ease his breathing and improve oxygenation.

♦ Give a diuretic to increase sodium and water elimination and reduce fluid overload.

 ALERT *Monitor the patient carefully during diuretic therapy because diuretics can disturb the electrolyte balance and lead to metabolic alkalosis, metabolic acidosis, or other complications.*

♦ Give an angiotensin-converting enzyme (ACE) inhibitor to decrease afterload and preload.

 ALERT *To prevent hyperkalemia in a patient receiving a potassium-sparing diuretic, discontinue diuretic therapy before beginning ACE inhibitor therapy.*

♦ Administer a beta-adrenergic blocker to decrease afterload and the heart's workload. Give a nitrate to dilate arterial smooth muscle.

♦ Give an inotropic drug such as digoxin to increase contractility and slow conduction through the atrioventricular node.

♦ Administer oral potassium in orange juice or with meals to promote absorption and prevent gastric irritation.

♦ Administer morphine for a patient who has acute pulmonary edema.

♦ Prepare the patient with severe heart failure for surgery if needed. For example, an intra-aortic balloon counterpulsation or other assist device may be implanted, or heart transplantation may be needed when other treatment options aren't possible.

♦ Monitor the patient's sodium and fluid intake.

♦ Provide continuous cardiac monitoring during the acute and advanced stages of heart failure.

Respiratory failure

◆ When the lungs can't sufficiently maintain arterial oxygenation or eliminate carbon dioxide (CO_2), acute respiratory failure results.

◆ If untreated, respiratory failure can lead to decreased oxygenation of the body tissues and fluid, electrolyte, and acid-base imbalances.

◆ Causes of respiratory failure include disorders of the brain, lungs, muscles and nerves, and pulmonary circulation.

◆ In acute respiratory failure, impaired gas exchange can result from any combination of these factors: alveolar hypoventilation, ventilation-perfusion mismatch, and intrapulmonary shunting.

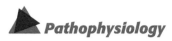

Pathophysiology

WHAT HAPPENS IN RESPIRATORY FAILURE

Three major malfunctions account for impaired gas exchange and subsequent acute respiratory failure: alveolar hypoventilation, ventilation-perfusion (V/Q) mismatch, and intrapulmonary (right-to-left) shunting.

Alveolar hypoventilation

In alveolar hypoventilation (shown below as the result of airway obstruction), the amount of oxygen brought to the alveoli is diminished, which causes a drop in the partial pressure of arterial oxygen and an increase in alveolar carbon dioxide (CO_2). The accumulation of CO_2 in the alveoli prevents diffusion of adequate amounts of CO_2 from the capillaries, which increases the partial pressure of arterial carbon dioxide.

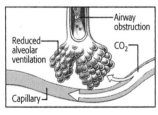

V/Q mismatch

V/Q mismatch, the leading cause of hypoxemia, occurs when insufficient ventilation exists with normal blood flow or when, as shown below, normal ventilation exists with insufficient blood flow. The Pao_2 is low, but the $Paco_2$ is normal because of normal ventilation in some parts of the lungs.

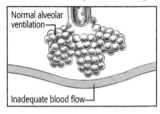

Intrapulmonary shunting

Intrapulmonary shunting occurs when blood passes from the right side of the heart to the left side without being oxygenated, as shown below. Shunting causes hypoxemia that doesn't respond to oxygen therapy.

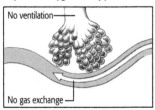

Causes

◆ Conditions affecting the brain.
- Anesthesia.
- Cerebral hemorrhage.
- Cerebral tumor.
- Drug overdose.
- Head trauma.
- Skull fracture.
◆ Lung disorders.
- Acute respiratory distress syndrome.
- Asthma.
- Chronic obstructive pulmonary disease (COPD).
- Cystic fibrosis.
- Flail chest.
- Massive bilateral pneumonia.
- Sleep apnea.
- Tracheal obstruction.
◆ Muscle and nerve disorders.
- Amyotrophic lateral sclerosis.
- Guillain-Barré syndrome.
- Multiple sclerosis.
- Muscular dystrophy.
- Myasthenia gravis.
- Polio.
- Spinal cord trauma.
◆ Pulmonary circulation problems.
- Heart failure.
- Pulmonary edema.
- Pulmonary embolism.

Imbalances caused by respiratory failure

◆ Hyperkalemia and hypokalemia.
◆ Hypervolemia and hypovolemia.
◆ Metabolic acidosis.
◆ Respiratory acidosis and alkalosis.

Signs and symptoms

◆ Increased heart rate.

◆ Increased respiratory depth and rate.

◆ Labored breathing with flared nostrils, pursed-lip exhalation, and the use of accessory breathing muscles.

◆ Muscle retractions between the ribs, above the clavicles, and above the sternum.

◆ Headache.

◆ Anxiety and restlessness, progressing to confusion, agitation, and lethargy.

◆ Cool, pale, clammy skin.

 ALERT *As respiratory failure worsens, be alert for arrhythmias, bradycardia, hypotension, cyanosis, dyspnea, diminished or absent breath sounds, wheezes, crackles, rhonchi, cardiac arrest, and respiratory arrest.*

Diagnostic test results

◆ Chest X-rays.
  – Evidence of a pulmonary disorder.

◆ ECG tracings.
  – Arrhythmias.

◆ Arterial blood gas (ABG) analysis.
  – Pao_2 level below 50 mm Hg (or below 10 mm Hg in a patient with COPD).
  – $Paco_2$ level above 50 mm Hg.
  – pH below 7.35 (SI, 7.35).

◆ Electrolyte levels.
  – Serum potassium level above or below normal.

Management

♦ Administer supplemental oxygen in a controlled concentration, for example, by using a Venturi mask.

 ALERT *Use caution when administering oxygen to a patient with COPD because an increased oxygen level can depress the breathing stimulus.*

♦ If conservative treatment doesn't raise the oxygen saturation above 90%, intubate the patient, and provide mechanical ventilation.

 ALERT *Avoid giving a narcotic or central nervous system (CNS) depressant to a patient who isn't mechanically ventilated because either drug may further suppress respirations.*

♦ Give a bronchodilator to open the airways.

♦ Administer a corticosteroid, a diuretic, and an antibiotic, as prescribed.

♦ Perform chest physiotherapy and postural drainage as needed to promote adequate ventilation.

♦ Suction if needed to clear the airways.

♦ Provide I.V. fluids to correct dehydration and to help thin secretions.

♦ Monitor and manage electrolyte and acid-base imbalances.

♦ Limit the patient's carbohydrate intake and increase his protein intake, because carbohydrate metabolism causes more CO_2 production than protein metabolism.

♦ Position the patient for maximum lung expansion. Sit the conscious patient upright as tolerated, in a supported, forward-leaning position.

♦ If the patient is retaining CO_2, encourage slow deep breaths with pursed lips. Urge him to cough up secretion.

Excessive GI fluid loss

◆ Significant fluid loss from the GI tract is possible because large amounts of fluids pass through the GI system daily.
◆ If fluid isn't reabsorbed in the intestines, isotonic fluid loss occurs.
◆ If saliva is lost, hypotonic fluid loss occurs.
◆ Excessive fluids can be excreted as waste products or secreted from the intestinal wall into the intestinal lumen. Either way, fluid and electrolyte imbalances can result.

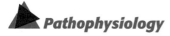 *Pathophysiology*

WHAT HAPPENS IN EXCESSIVE GI FLUID LOSS

GI fluid loss results from vomiting, suctioning, or altered GI motility.

⬇

Hypovolemia occurs.

⬇

To compensate, heart rate increases.

⬇

Tachycardia and hypotension occur as intravascular volume diminishes.

⬇

Body shunts blood to major organs, causing cool, dry skin.

⬇

Urine output and skin turgor decrease, and eyeballs appear sunken.

⬇

Electrolyte imbalances and arrhythmias cause weakness and confusion.

⬇

Patient's mental status deteriorates.

Causes

- ◆ Physical removal of secretions.
  - – Vomiting.
  - – Suctioning.
  - – Increased or decreased GI tract motility.
- ◆ Other causes.
  - – Anorexia nervosa or bulimia.
  - – Antibiotic use.
  - – Bacterial infection.
  - – Enema or laxative use.
  - – Enteral tube feedings and ostomies.
  - – Excessive intake of alcohol or illicit drugs.
  - – Hepatitis or pancreatitis.
  - – Poor absorption or digestion.
  - – Pregnancy.
  - – Pyloric stenosis in young children.
  - – Young age.

 AGE ALERT *Young children are particularly vulnerable to fluid loss from diarrhea.*

Imbalances caused by excessive GI fluid loss

- ◆ Dehydration and hypovolemia.
- ◆ Hypochloremia.
- ◆ Hypokalemia.
- ◆ Hypomagnesemia.
- ◆ Hyponatremia.
- ◆ Metabolic acidosis and alkalosis.

Signs and symptoms

◆ Decreased blood pressure.
◆ Arrhythmias and tachycardia.
◆ Increased heart rate.
◆ Altered respirations.
◆ Decreased urine output.
◆ Decreased skin turgor and sunken eyeballs.
◆ Cool, dry skin.
◆ Confusion and weakness.

 AGE ALERT *When assessing an adolescent, especially a girl, for excessive GI fluid loss, check for signs and symptoms of anorexia and bulimia. Teeth that appear yellow and worn away, and a history of laxative and diet pill use are two obvious signs.*

Diagnostic test results

◆ ABG analysis.
– Levels that reflect metabolic acidosis or alkalosis.
◆ Electrolyte levels.
– Altered levels of certain electrolytes, notably potassium, magnesium, and sodium.
◆ Other blood tests.
– Falsely elevated hematocrit (HCT).
◆ Other tests.
– Cultures of body fluid samples that identify the bacteria causing the infection.

Management

◆ Monitor for an increase in the amount of drainage from GI tubes, an increase in suctioning, or an increase in the frequency of vomiting or diarrhea.

◆ Assess the patient's fluid status by monitoring intake and output, daily weight, and skin turgor.

◆ Administer oral fluids that contain water and electrolytes, such as Gatorade or Pedialyte.

◆ Administer I.V. replacement fluids, using an infusion pump to prevent hypervolemia.

◆ If the patient is undergoing gastric suctioning, frequently check GI tube placement to prevent fluid aspiration.

◆ Irrigate the suction tube with isotonic normal saline solution.

 ALERT *Never use plain water for irrigation. It draws more gastric secretions into the stomach in an attempt to make the fluid isotonic for absorption.*

◆ When the patient is connected to gastric suction, restrict the amount of ice chips given by mouth because gastric suctioning of ice chips can deplete fluid and electrolytes from the stomach.

◆ Give drugs, such as an antiemetic or antidiarrheal, to treat the underlying condition as prescribed.

◆ Evaluate serum electrolyte levels and pH.

Renal failure

- Renal failure involves a disruption of normal kidney function and may be acute or chronic.
- Acute renal failure occurs suddenly and is often reversible. Chronic renal failure occurs slowly and is irreversible.
- Both types of renal failure affect renal function, producing imbalances as the kidneys lose the ability to excrete water, electrolytes, wastes, and acid-base products in urine.
- Causes of acute renal failure may be prerenal, intrarenal, or postrenal.
- Chronic renal failure develops in four stages: reduced renal reserve (glomerular filtration rate [GFR] 40 to 70 ml/min), renal insufficiency (GFR 20 to 40 ml/min), renal failure (GFR 10 to 20 ml/min), and end-stage renal disease (GFR less than 10 ml/min).

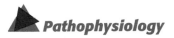

Pathophysiology

WHAT HAPPENS IN RENAL FAILURE

Acute renal failure	Chronic renal failure
Kidneys sustain damage, urine flow is obstructed, or renal blood flow diminishes.	Kidney function deteriorates gradually. Eventually, more than 75% of glomerular filtration is lost.
Glomerular filtration rate (GFR) decreases.	Patient develops symptoms of uremia. Kidneys can no longer regulate fluid, electrolyte, and acid-base balance. Uremic toxins accumulate.
Urine output falls to less than 400 ml in 24 hours.	Patient needs renal transplantation or dialysis.
Kidneys fail.	
Nitrogenous waste products accumulate.	
Blood urea nitrogen (BUN) and serum creatinine levels rise.	
Uremia occurs.	
Uremia causes electrolyte imbalances, metabolic acidosis, and hypervolemia, as renal dysfunction disrupts other body systems.	

Causes

Acute renal failure

◆ Prerenal causes.
  – Serious cardiovascular disorders.
  – Hypovolemia.
  – Peripheral vasodilation.
  – Severe vasoconstriction.
  – Renal vascular obstruction.
  – Trauma.
◆ Intrarenal causes.
  – Acute tubular necrosis.
  – Exposure to nephrotoxins or heavy metals.
  – Use of aminoglycosides or nonsteroidal anti-inflammatory drugs.
  – Ischemic damage from poorly treated renal failure.
  – Eclampsia.
  – Postpartum renal failure.
  – Uterine hemorrhage.
  – Crush injury.
  – Myopathy.
  – Sepsis.
  – Transfusion reaction.
  – Trauma.
◆ Postrenal causes.
  – Obstruction of the bladder, ureters, or urethra.
  – Trauma.

Chronic renal failure

  – Chronic glomerular disease.
  – Chronic infection.
  – Congenital anomaly.
  – Vascular disease.
  – Obstruction (as with calculi).
  – Collagen disease.
  – Long-term nephrotoxic drug therapy.
  – Endocrine disease.

Imbalances caused by renal failure

- ◆ Hyperkalemia.
- ◆ Hypermagnesemia.
- ◆ Hypernatremia and hyponatremia.
- ◆ Hyperphosphatemia.
- ◆ Hypervolemia and hypovolemia.
- ◆ Hypocalcemia.
- ◆ Metabolic acidosis and alkalosis.

Signs and symptoms

Neurologic

◆ Burning, itching, and pain in the legs and feet.
◆ Muscle irritability, twitching, and tremors.
◆ Seizures.
◆ Shortened attention span and memory.
◆ Confusion.
◆ Irritability.
◆ Listlessness and somnolence.
◆ Fatigue.
◆ Coma.
◆ Hiccups.

Cardiovascular

◆ Arrhythmias.
◆ Hypertension or hypotension.
◆ Irregular pulse.
◆ Tachycardia.
◆ Pericardial rub.
◆ Heart failure.
◆ Anemia.
◆ Weight gain with fluid retention.

Pulmonary

◆ Dyspnea.
◆ Crackles.
◆ Decreased breath sounds, if pneumonia is present.
◆ Kussmaul's respirations.

GI

◆ Nausea and vomiting.
◆ Metallic taste.
◆ Dry mouth.
◆ Inflammation and ulceration of GI mucosa.
◆ Constipation or diarrhea.
◆ Anorexia.
◆ Bleeding.
◆ Pain on abdominal palpation and percussion.
◆ Ammonia breath odor.

Integumentary

◆ Severe itching.

◆ Loss of skin turgor.

◆ Dry, scaly skin with ecchymoses, petechiae, and purpura.

◆ Dry mucous membranes.

◆ Dry, brittle hair that may change color or fall out easily.

◆ Thin, brittle fingernails with lines.

◆ Yellow-bronze skin color.

◆ Uremic frost (in later stages).

Genitourinary

◆ Anuria or oliguria.

◆ Changes in urinary appearance or patterns.

◆ Dilute urine with casts and crystals.

◆ Amenorrhea in women.

◆ Infertility.

◆ Impotence in men.

◆ Decreased libido.

Musculoskeletal

◆ Muscle weakness.

◆ Muscle cramps.

◆ Bone and muscle pain.

◆ Gait abnormalities.

◆ Pathologic fractures.

◆ Inability to ambulate.

Diagnostic test results

◆ ABG analysis.
  – Changes that indicate metabolic acidosis.
  – Low pH.
  – Low bicarbonate level.
◆ ECG tracings.
  – Tall, peaked T waves.
  – Widened QRS complexes.
  – Disappearing P waves, if hyperkalemia is present.
◆ Electrolyte levels.
  – Elevated potassium and phosphorus levels.
◆ Other blood tests.
  – Elevated blood urea nitrogen (BUN) and serum creatinine.

 AGE ALERT *As people age, nephrons are lost and kidneys decrease in size. These physiologic changes decrease renal blood flow and may result in doubled BUN levels in older patients.*

  – Low HCT.
  – Low hemoglobin (Hb) level.
  – Mild thrombocytopenia.
◆ Urinalysis.
  – Casts.
  – Cellular debris.
  – Decreased specific gravity.
  – Proteinuria.

Management

◆ Provide a low-protein, high-calorie diet and restrict the patient's intake of potassium, sodium, phosphorus, and fluid.

◆ Give a diuretic only if the patient has some degree of renal function.

◆ Monitor the patient's serum electrolyte and ABG levels. If imbalances occur, intervene appropriately.

◆ If the patient is anemic, administer iron and synthetic erythropoietin and provide blood transfusions as indicated.

◆ Administer a phosphorus-binding drug with meals to decrease the phosphorus level.

◆ Monitor for ECG changes to help detect electrolyte imbalances.

◆ Monitor the Hb level and HCT.

◆ Give sodium bicarbonate I.V. if needed to control acute acidosis.

 ALERT *Remember that sodium bicarbonate has a high sodium content and that multiple doses may result in hypernatremia, which could contribute to the onset of heart failure and pulmonary edema.*

◆ Begin dialysis to manage hypervolemia and electrolyte and acid-base imbalances. If the patient is hemodynamically unstable, provide continuous renal replacement therapy in the critical care setting.

◆ Frequently assess the hemodialysis access site for patency, bleeding, and signs of infection.

 ALERT *Never use the arm with a hemodialysis graft or fistula for measuring blood pressure, drawing blood, or inserting I.V. catheters. These actions could compromise the hemodialysis access site, which is the patient's connection for a life-sustaining therapy.*

◆ Check the route of excretion for drugs and adjust their dosages as needed.

Syndrome of inappropriate antidiuretic hormone secretion

◆ Syndrome of inappropriate antidiuretic hormone (SIADH) secretion causes an excessive release of antidiuretic hormone (ADH) and disturbs fluid and electrolyte balance.
◆ ADH is released when the body doesn't need it, which results in water retention and sodium excretion.

 Pathophysiology

WHAT HAPPENS IN SIADH

The body secretes too much antidiuretic hormone (ADH).

⬇

ADH increases renal tubule permeability.

⬇

Increased tubule permeability increases water retention and extracellular fluid (ECF) volume.

⬇

Increased ECF volume leads to:

⬇ ⬇ ⬇ ⬇

Reduced plasma osmolality.	Dilutional hyponatremia.	Diminished aldosterone secretion.	Elevated glomerular filtration rate.

⬇ ⬇

Sodium excretion increases, and fluid shifts into cells.

Patient develops thirst, dyspnea on exertion, vomiting, abdominal cramps, confusion, lethargy, and hyponatremia.

Causes

◆ Cancers.
◆ CNS disorders.
◆ Pulmonary disorders.
◆ Use of certain drugs.
   – Some oral antidiabetics.
   – Chemotherapeutic drugs.
   – Psychoactive drugs.
   – Diuretics.
   – Synthetic hormones.
   – Barbiturates.

Imbalances caused by SIADH

◆ Hypervolemia.
◆ Isovolumic hyponatremia.

Signs and symptoms

◆ Nausea and vomiting.
◆ Anorexia.
◆ Abdominal cramps.
◆ Muscle twitching, tremors, and weakness.
◆ Confusion.
◆ Headache.
◆ Lethargy.
◆ Seizures, stupor, and coma.

Diagnostic test results

◆ Electrolyte levels.
  – Serum sodium level below 135 mEq/L (SI, 135 mmol/L).
◆ Other blood tests.
  – Elevated HCT and plasma protein levels.
  – Serum osmolality less than 280 mOsm/kg.
◆ Urine tests.
  – Urine specific gravity above normal.
  – Urine sodium level above 20 mEq/L (SI, 20 mmol/L).

Management

◆ Restrict the patient's fluid intake to 500 to 1,000 ml/day.
◆ Consider a high-sodium, high-protein diet or urea supplements to enhance fluid excretion.
◆ Administer demeclocycline or lithium to block the renal response to ADH.
◆ Give a loop diuretic to prevent heart failure.
◆ Infuse a hypertonic saline solution to replace lost sodium.
◆ Elevate the head of the bed to promote venous return. (Decreased venous return is a stimulus for ADH release.)
◆ Monitor the serum sodium level and adjust the flow rate of the I.V. saline infusion accordingly.

 ALERT *A serum sodium level that rises too quickly puts the patient at risk for neurologic damage. Therefore, increase the serum sodium level by less than 12 mEq/L (SI, 12 mmol/L) in 24 hours.*

◆ Correct the underlying cause of SIADH.

Burns

◆ A burn interferes with the skin's ability to help keep out infectious organisms, maintain fluid balance, and regulate body temperature.

◆ Burns can result from thermal, mechanical, or electrical injuries as well as from exposure to chemicals or radiation.

◆ First-degree (partial-thickness) burns affect the superficial layer of the epidermis.

◆ Second-degree (deep partial-thickness) burns affect the epidermis and dermis.

◆ Third-degree (full-thickness) burns affect the epidermis, dermis, and underlying tissues.

◆ The extent of a burn can be estimated with a tool, such as the Rule of Nines or the Lund-Browder chart. (See *Estimating the Extent of a Burn,* pages 150 and 151.)

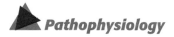

Pathophysiology

WHAT HAPPENS IN BURNS

Burn injury occurs.

▼

Capillary damage alters vessel permeability.
(Fluid accumulation phase begins.)

▼

Plasma escapes from intravascular space into interstitial space
(third-space shift). Blood becomes hemoconcentrated, causing hemoglobin
and hematocrit to increase.

▼

Third-space shift leads to hypovolemia.

▼

Hypovolemia decreases cardiac output and causes tachycardia
and hypotension.

▼

Diminished kidney perfusion decreases urine output, and the body releases
aldosterone and antidiuretic hormone (ADH) as a result of stress and the
body's response to burns.

▼

Aldosterone and ADH prompt kidneys to retain sodium and water, and
injured tissue releases acids, causing metabolic acidosis.

▼

Patient may develop fluid and electrolyte imbalances.

ESTIMATING THE EXTENT OF A BURN

You can quickly estimate the extent of an *adult* patient's burns by using the Rule of Nines (below). This method divides an adult's body surface into percentages.

To use this method, match your adult patient's burns to the body chart shown here. Then add up the corresponding percentages for each burned section. The total—a rough estimate of the extent of your patient's burns—enters into the formula to determine his initial fluid replacement needs.

An infant or a child's body-surface percentages differ from those of an adult. For instance, an infant's head accounts for a greater percentage of his total body surface when compared with an adult's. For an *infant* or *child,* use the Lund-Browder chart (at right).

Rule of Nines

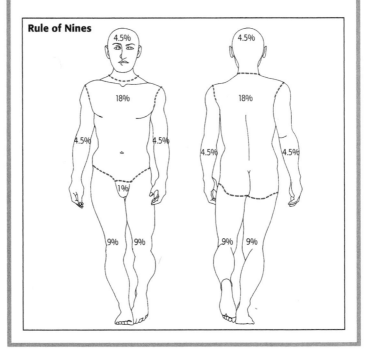

ESTIMATING THE EXTENT OF A BURN *(continued)*

Lund-Browder chart

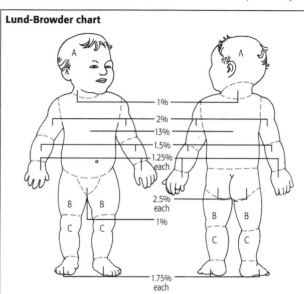

Relative percentages of areas affected by growth

	At birth	1–4 yr	5–9 yr	10–14 yr	15 yr	Adult
A: Half of head						
	9.5%	8.5%	6.5%	5.5%	4.5%	3.5%
B: Half of thigh						
	2.75%	3.25%	4%	4.25%	4.5%	4.75%
C: Half of leg						
	2.5%	2.5%	2.75%	3%	3.25%	3.5%

Causes

◆ Thermal injuries.
  – Exposure to dry heat (flames).
  – Exposure to moist heat (steam or hot liquids).
◆ Mechanical injuries.
  – Friction or abrasion from skin rubbing harshly against a coarse surface.
◆ Electrical injuries.
  – Contact with high-voltage power lines.
  – Immersion in water that has been electrified.
  – Lightning strikes.
◆ Chemical and radiation burns.
  – Direct contact, ingestion, inhalation, or injection of acids, alkali, or vesicants.

Imbalances caused by burns

◆ Hyperkalemia and hypokalemia.
◆ Hypernatremia and hyponatremia.
◆ Hypervolemia and hypovolemia.
◆ Hypocalcemia.
◆ Metabolic acidosis.
◆ Respiratory acidosis.

Signs and symptoms

First-degree burns

◆ Burns of the epidermis only.

◆ Dry, painful wound.

◆ Pink or red appearance.

◆ Slight edema.

Second-degree burns

◆ Burns of the epidermis and dermis.

◆ Painful wound.

◆ Swollen, red appearance.

◆ Blisters.

◆ Blanching and refill when pressure is applied.

◆ Variable amount of scarring.

Third-degree burns

◆ Burns of the epidermis, dermis, and tissues below the dermis.

◆ Painless wound.

◆ White to black (charred) color.

◆ Dry, leathery appearance.

◆ No blanching when pressure is applied.

Diagnostic test results

- ◆ ABG analysis.
  - – Bicarbonate level below normal.
  - – pH below normal.
- ◆ Electrolyte levels.
  - – Serum potassium level above normal.
  - – Serum sodium level below normal.
- ◆ Other blood tests.
  - – BUN and creatinine levels above normal.
  - – Carboxyhemoglobin level above normal.
  - – Hb level and HCT above normal.
- ◆ ECG tracings.
  - – Changes characteristic of electrolyte imbalances or myocardial damage.
- ◆ Urine tests.
  - – Myoglobin in urine.

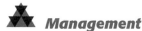 *Management*

Emergency burn care

◆ Extinguish any remaining flames on the patient's clothing.
◆ Don't directly touch the patient if he's still connected to live electricity. Unplug or disconnect the electrical source if possible.
◆ Assess the ABCs (airway, breathing, and circulation) and begin cardiopulmonary resuscitation, if needed.
◆ Assess the scope of the burns and other injuries.
◆ Remove the patient's clothing, but don't pull at clothing that sticks to the skin.
◆ Irrigate areas of chemical burns with copious amounts of water.
◆ Remove from the patient any jewelry or other metal objects that can retain heat and constrict patient movement.
◆ Cover the patient with a blanket.
◆ Send for emergency medical assistance.

Continuing burn care

◆ Treat severe facial burns or inhalation injuries with intubation, administration of high concentrations of oxygen, and positive-pressure ventilation.
◆ Provide initial fluid resuscitation with lactated Ringer's solution.

FLUID REPLACEMENT FORMULA

Here's a commonly used formula, the Parkland formula, for calculating fluid replacement in burn patients. Vary volumes of infusions depending on the patient's response, especially his urine output.

Formula

4 ml of lactated Ringer's solution/kg of body weight/% of body surface area (BSA) over 24 hours.

Example

For a 68-kg person with 27% BSA burns:
4 ml × 68 kg × 27 = 7,344 ml over 24 hours.
Give one-half of the total over the first 8 hours after the burn and the remainder over the next 16 hours.

◆ Administer colloids if prescribed to increase blood volume.

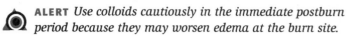 **ALERT** *Use colloids cautiously in the immediate postburn period because they may worsen edema at the burn site.*

◆ Infuse dextrose 5% in water solution to replace normal insensible water loss and losses caused by damage to the skin barrier. (If needed, add potassium to I.V. solutions 48 to 72 hours after the burn.)

◆ Insert a nasogastric tube to prevent gastric distention from paralytic ileus.

◆ Give an I.M. booster of tetanus toxoid.

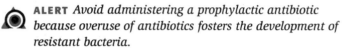 **ALERT** *Avoid administering a prophylactic antibiotic because overuse of antibiotics fosters the development of resistant bacteria.*

◆ Debride the wound. Assist with an escharotomy to prevent burn-induced compartment syndrome.

◆ Monitor for fluid, electrolyte, and acid-base imbalances.

◆ Give an analgesic 30 minutes before wound care. Use biological dressings for full-thickness burns and non-biological dressings for partial-thickness burns.

◆ Maintain joint function with physical therapy and the use of splints and support garments.

◆ If bowel sounds are present, provide a diet high in potassium, protein, vitamins, fats, nitrogen, and calories. Provide enteral or parenteral nutrition if the patient can't tolerate oral intake.

6

Treating imbalances

A look at treatments

- ◆ Depending on the type of imbalance and the patient's condition, treatment may require I.V. fluids, total parenteral nutrition (TPN), dialysis, or transfusion of blood or blood products.
- ◆ Although each treatment corrects imbalances, it can lead to complications and requires expert clinical management.

I.V. replacement therapy

◆ I.V. therapy provides the patient with life-sustaining fluids, electrolytes, and drugs.

◆ Advantages of I.V. therapy include immediate and predictable therapeutic effects, provision of fluid for a patient with GI malabsorption, and accurate I.V. drug titration.

◆ Disadvantages of I.V. therapy include drug and solution incompatibility, adverse reactions, and infection and other complications.

◆ Solutions for I.V. therapy fall into the broad categories of crystalloids (which may be isotonic, hypertonic, or hypotonic) and colloids (which are always hypertonic).

◆ Crystalloids are solutions with small molecules that flow easily from the bloodstream into cells and tissues.

◆ Colloids are solutions with larger molecules used to expand plasma.

Isotonic solutions

◆ Isotonic solutions have a concentration of dissolved particles (tonicity) equal to the intracellular fluid, so fluid doesn't shift between the extracellular and intracellular spaces.

◆ With isotonic solutions, the osmotic pressure is the same inside and outside cells.

◆ Cells neither shrink nor swell with isotonic fluid movement.

◆ Examples of isotonic solutions include dextrose 5% in water (D_5W), normal saline (0.9% sodium chloride), and lactated Ringer's solutions.

◆ Different isotonic solutions have different uses and special considerations.

Dextrose 5% in water solution

Uses

◆ Fluid loss and dehydration.

◆ Hypernatremia.

 ALERT *Use D_5W solution cautiously in patients with renal or cardiac disease because it can cause fluid overload.*

Special considerations

◆ Remember that D_5W solution is isotonic initially and then becomes hypotonic when dextrose is metabolized.

 ALERT *Don't use D_5W solution for resuscitation because it can cause hyperglycemia.*

◆ This solution doesn't provide enough daily calories for prolonged use and eventually may cause protein breakdown.

Normal saline solution

Uses

◆ Blood transfusion.
◆ Fluid challenge.
◆ Fluid replacement in patients with diabetic ketoacidosis (DKA).
◆ Hypercalcemia.
◆ Hyponatremia.
◆ Metabolic alkalosis.
◆ Resuscitation.
◆ Shock.

Special considerations

◆ Consider normal saline solution as a replacement for extracellular fluid (ECF).
◆ Don't use it in patients with heart failure, edema, or hypernatremia because it can lead to fluid overload.

Lactated Ringer's solution

Uses

◆ Acute blood loss.
◆ Burns.
◆ Dehydration.
◆ Hypovolemia caused by third-space shifting.
◆ Lower GI tract fluid loss.

Special considerations

◆ The electrolyte content of lactated Ringer's solution is similar to that of serum, but it doesn't contain magnesium.
◆ Because this solution contains potassium, don't use it in patients with renal failure; otherwise, hyperkalemia can occur.
◆ Don't use lactated Ringer's solution in liver disease because the patient can't metabolize the lactate.
◆ Don't use this solution in a patient whose pH exceeds 7.5 (SI, 7.5).

Hypertonic solutions

◆ Hypertonic solutions have greater tonicity than intracellular fluid.

◆ In hypertonic solutions, the osmotic pressure is unequal inside and outside cells.

◆ Hypertonic solutions draw water out of cells into ECF.

◆ Examples of hypertonic solutions include dextrose 5% in half-normal saline, dextrose 5% in normal saline, dextrose 5% in lactated Ringer's, and dextrose 10% in water.

◆ Different hypertonic solutions have different uses and special considerations.

Dextrose 5% in half-normal saline solution

Uses

◆ DKA after initial treatment with normal saline solution and half-normal saline solution.

◆ Prevention of hypoglycemia and cerebral edema in DKA treatment.

Special considerations

◆ In a patient with DKA, use this solution only when the glucose level falls below 250 mg/dl (SI, 13.9 mmol/L).

Dextrose 5% in normal saline solution

Uses

◆ Addisonian crisis.

◆ Hypotonic dehydration.

◆ Syndrome of inappropriate antidiuretic hormone (SIADH) secretion.

◆ Temporary treatment of circulatory insufficiency and shock if plasma expanders aren't available.

Special considerations

◆ Don't use this solution in cardiac or renal patients because of the danger of heart failure and pulmonary edema.

Dextrose 10% in water solution

Uses

◆ Conditions in which some nutrition with glucose is required.

◆ Water replacement.

Special considerations

◆ Monitor the patient's serum glucose level during therapy with dextrose 10% in water solution.

Hypotonic solutions

◆ Hypotonic solutions have less tonicity than intracellular fluid.
◆ In hypotonic solutions, the osmotic pressure pulls water into cells from ECF.
◆ Cellular swelling results from hypotonic fluid therapy.
◆ Examples of hypertonic solutions include half-normal saline (0.45% sodium chloride), 0.33% sodium chloride, and dextrose 2.5% in water solutions.
◆ Different hypotonic solutions have different uses and special considerations.

Half-normal saline solution

Uses

◆ DKA after initial treatment with normal saline solution and before dextrose infusion.
◆ Gastric fluid loss from nasogastric suctioning or vomiting.
◆ Hypertonic dehydration.
◆ Sodium and chloride depletion.
◆ Water replacement.

Special considerations

◆ Use half-normal saline solution cautiously because it may cause cardiovascular collapse or increased intracranial pressure (ICP).
◆ Don't use this solution in a patient with liver disease, trauma, or burns.

Colloid solutions

Types
◆ Albumin.
◆ Dextran.
◆ Hetastarch.
◆ Plasma protein factor.

Uses
◆ Expansion of plasma in patients who don't respond to crystalloids.
◆ Improvement of microcirculation.

Special considerations
◆ Be aware that the effects of colloids may last several days.
◆ During colloid infusion, monitor the patient for signs of hypervolemia, such as increased blood pressure, dyspnea, and bounding pulses.

Complications of I.V. therapy

◆ I.V. therapy requires careful patient monitoring and an ability to detect and properly deal with complications and flow issues.

◆ The most common complications of I.V. therapy are infiltration, infection, phlebitis, and thrombophlebitis.

◆ Other complications include extravasation, a severed catheter, an allergic reaction, an air embolism, speed shock, and fluid overload.

Infiltration

In infiltration, non-vesicant fluid leaks from the vein into surrounding tissue. This complication occurs when an I.V. access device becomes dislodged from a vein.

Signs and symptoms

◆ Pain, swelling, and leakage.

◆ Coolness at the site.

◆ Sluggish flow even when a tourniquet is placed above the site.

◆ Peripheral nerve damage (with a large infiltrate).

Management

◆ Stop the infusion.

◆ Elevate the arm or leg.

◆ Remove the catheter and restart in another site in the other extremity.

Prevention

◆ Use the smallest catheter to accommodate the infusion.

◆ Avoid catheter placement in joint areas.

◆ Anchor the catheter in place.

◆ Consider using a gravity drip rather than an I.V. pump for a small I.V. catheter in a small vein.

Infection

Infection occurs because the puncture for venous access disrupts the integrity of the skin, the body's barrier to infection.

Signs and symptoms

◆ Drainage, tenderness, redness, and warmth at the I.V. site.
◆ Hardness on palpation.
◆ Fever and chills.
◆ Elevated white blood cell (WBC) count.

Management

◆ Monitor the patient's vital signs and notify the physician.
◆ Swab the site for culture and sensitivity testing.
◆ Remove the catheter as ordered.

Prevention

◆ Maintain sterile technique.
◆ Consider using a chlorhexidine antiseptic wipe or foam-impregnated disc for site care in a patient with a central line.
◆ Change catheter hubs routinely.
◆ Rotate peripheral I.V. catheter sites every 72 hours.

Phlebitis and thrombophlebitis

Phlebitis is an inflammation of the vein and can be mechanical, chemical, or bacterial. Thrombophlebitis is an irritation of the vein with clot formation. Phlebitis and thrombophlebitis can result from poor insertion technique, use of a solution or drug with an inappropriate pH or osmolality, or a peripheral I.V. catheter remaining in place too long.

Signs and symptoms

- Pain (more severe in thrombophlebitis), redness, swelling, or induration at the site.
- Red line streaking along the vein.
- Sluggish flow of the infusing solution.
- Fever.

Management

- Remove the I.V.
- Monitor the patient's vital signs and notify the physician.
- Apply warm soaks to the site.

Prevention

- Choose large bore veins.
- Change the catheter every 72 hours when infusing a drug or solution with high osmolality.
- Treat a central line occlusion with a fibrinolytic.
- Flush the catheter exactly as directed in facility protocol.
- Dilute the drug and infuse at a slower rate.

Extravasation

Extravasation is the leakage of vesicant fluid into surrounding tissue. It results when drugs seep through veins and produce blistering and necrosis.

Signs and symptoms

- Discomfort, stinging, and burning at the infusion site (initially).
- Skin tightness, blanching, and lack of blood return.
- Inflammation and pain (in 3 to 5 days).
- Ulcers and necrosis (in 2 weeks).

Management

- Stop the infusion and notify the physician.
- Infiltrate the site with an antidote as prescribed.
- Apply ice to the I.V. site initially, followed by warm soaks.
- Elevate the affected arm or leg.
- Assess the circulation and nerve function of the affected limb.

Prevention

- Follow facility policy when giving drugs that may extravasate.

Severed catheter

A severed catheter occurs when a piece of catheter becomes dislodged and is set free in the vein. It can result from defective equipment or poor insertion technique. This complication is extremely rare but serious.

Signs and symptoms
- Pain at the fragment site.
- Weak, rapid pulses.
- Cyanosis.
- Decreased blood pressure.
- Loss of consciousness.

Management
- Apply a tourniquet above the site of pain.
- Notify the physician immediately.
- Monitor the patient.

Prevention
- Avoid reinserting a needle through its plastic catheter once the needle has been withdrawn.
- Pull PICC lines out slowly, and never pull hard against resistance.

Allergic reaction

A patient may suffer an allergic reaction to a fluid, drug, I.V. catheter, or latex in the tubing. However, the source of the reaction may not be known. If untreated, an allergic reaction may lead to anaphylaxis.

Signs and symptoms

◆ Red streak up the arm.
◆ Rash and itching.
◆ Watery eyes and nose.
◆ Wheezing.

Management

◆ Stop the I.V. infusion immediately.
◆ Notify the physician.
◆ Give supplemental oxygen and drugs, as prescribed.

Prevention

◆ Check the patient's record for allergies and hypersensitivity reactions.

Air embolism

An air embolism occurs when air enters the vein. This complication can result from inadvertent injection or infusion of an air bubble along with the fluid or drug. It's more likely to occur in central lines than in peripheral lines that enter veins above the level of the heart.

Signs and symptoms
- Increased pulse rate.
- Decreased blood pressure.
- Respiratory distress.
- Increased ICP.
- Loss of consciousness.

Management
- Clamp off the I.V. line.
- Notify the physician immediately.
- Place patient on his left side in Trendelenburg's position. This position allows air to enter the right atrium, where it can be removed more easily by the pulmonary artery.

Prevention
- Prime all tubing completely.
- Tighten all connections securely.
- Use an air detection device on the I.V. pump.

Speed shock

Speed shock is a systemic reaction that occurs when a substance is introduced into the circulation at a rapid rate. This complication commonly occurs when an I.V. solution or drug is given too quickly.

Signs and symptoms

◆ Decreased blood pressure.

◆ Irregular pulse.

◆ Facial flushing.

◆ Severe headache.

◆ Loss of consciousness and cardiac arrest.

Management

◆ Clamp off the I.V. line immediately.

◆ Notify the physician immediately.

◆ Provide supplemental oxygen.

Prevention

◆ Use an infusion control device.

Fluid overload

Fluid overload can occur gradually or suddenly, depending on the patient's circulatory system and the ability to accommodate fluid.

Signs and symptoms

◆ Increased blood pressure.
◆ Neck vein distention.
◆ Increased respirations.
◆ Shortness of breath.
◆ Crackles on auscultation.
◆ Cough.

Management

◆ Slow the I.V. infusion rate.
◆ Notify the physician and monitor the patient's vital signs.
◆ Keep the patient warm.
◆ Elevate the head of the bed.
◆ Give supplemental oxygen and drugs, as prescribed.

Prevention

◆ Always use an infusion pump to administer solutions.
◆ Always clamp the catheter when changing the I.V. solution.
◆ Consider the patient's size and age, and adjust fluid administration as needed.

Total parenteral nutrition

- TPN is a highly concentrated, hypertonic nutrient solution administered by infusion pump through a large central vein.
- TPN provides crucial calories, restores nitrogen balance, and replaces fluids, vitamins, electrolytes, minerals, and trace elements.
- TPN must be administered through a central vein.
- Peripheral parenteral nutrition is a combination of lipids and amino acid-dextrose solution; it may be infused peripherally for less than 7 days.

Uses

- Debilitating illness lasting longer than 2 weeks.
- Loss of 10% or more of pre-illness weight.
- Serum albumin level below 3.5 g/dl (SI, 35 g/L).
- Excessive nitrogen loss from a wound infection, fistula, or abscess.
- Renal or hepatic failure.
- Nonfunction of the GI tract lasting for 5 to 7 days.

Common TPN additives

◆ Substances such as electrolytes and vitamins are commonly added to TPN for specific purposes.

◆ Lipids may be added to TPN or infused separately.

Electrolytes

◆ Calcium promotes the development of bones and teeth, and aids in blood clotting.

◆ Chloride regulates acid-base balance, and maintains osmotic pressure.

◆ Magnesium helps the body absorb carbohydrates and protein.

◆ Phosphorus is essential for cell energy and calcium balance.

◆ Potassium is needed for cellular activity and cardiac function.

◆ Sodium helps control water distribution, and maintains normal fluid balance.

Vitamins

◆ Folic acid is needed for deoxyribonucleic acid formation and promotes growth and development.

◆ Vitamin A is a fat-soluble vitamin that's necessary for cell and bone growth.

◆ Vitamin B complex helps the final absorption of carbohydrates and protein.

◆ Vitamin C aids in wound healing.

◆ Vitamin D is essential for bone metabolism and maintenance of the serum calcium level.

◆ Vitamin E is a fat-soluble vitamin that acts as an antioxidant to help protect cells from damage caused by the body's by-products of metabolism.

◆ Vitamin K helps prevent bleeding disorders.

Other additives

◆ Acetate prevents metabolic acidosis.

◆ Amino acids provide the proteins needed for tissue repair.

◆ Micronutrients, such as zinc, chromium, selenium, and copper, help in wound healing and red blood cell (RBC) synthesis.

◆ Drugs, such as insulin, to manage hyperglycemia related to concentrated dextrose infusion.

Lipid emulsions

◆ Lipid emulsions supply patients with essential fatty acids and calories.

◆ These thick emulsions usually are given with TPN but may be given alone via a peripheral or central venous line.

◆ They assist in wound healing, RBC production, and prostaglandin synthesis.

◆ These emulsions shouldn't be given to patients who have conditions that disrupt normal fat metabolism, such as pathologic hyperlipidemia, lipid nephrosis, and acute pancreatitis.

◆ Adverse reactions to lipid emulsions may be immediate (or early) or delayed (with prolonged administration).

ADVERSE REACTIONS TO LIPID EMULSIONS

Immediate reactions
◆ Back and chest pain.
◆ Cyanosis.
◆ Diaphoresis or flushing.
◆ Dyspnea.
◆ Headache.
◆ Irritation at the site.
◆ Lethargy or syncope.
◆ Nausea and vomiting.
◆ Thrombocytopenia.

Delayed reactions
◆ Fatty liver syndrome.
◆ Hepatomegaly.
◆ Jaundice.
◆ Splenomegaly.

Complications of TPN

◆ Acid-base imbalances.
◆ Electrolyte imbalances, with such effects as abdominal cramps, arrhythmias, confusion, lethargy, malaise, muscle weakness, seizures, and tetany.
◆ Heart failure or pulmonary edema.
◆ Hyperglycemia.
◆ Hypoglycemia if insulin is added to the TPN solution.
◆ Infection or sepsis.
◆ I.V. cannula and central venous catheter complications.
◆ Liver dysfunction.

Care related to TPN

◆ Infuse TPN around the clock or for part of the day (usually at night), as prescribed.

◆ Use a silicone rubber (Silastic) catheter, which is preferred because it's more flexible and durable than other catheters and is compatible with many drugs and solutions.

◆ For therapy lasting 3 months or more, use a peripherally inserted central catheter.

◆ Weigh the patient daily to assess his nutritional progress and to detect fluid overload. Also assess for edema, a sign of fluid overload.

◆ Monitor the serum glucose level at least every 6 hours. Add insulin to the TPN solution as prescribed.

◆ When TPN begins, monitor the electrolyte and protein levels daily.

◆ Assess the patient's nitrogen balance with a 24-hour urine collection.

◆ Initiate TPN or a lipid emulsion slowly, and monitor for adverse reactions. With TPN, also monitor for signs and symptoms of hyperglycemia.

◆ Monitor for signs of refeeding syndrome, such as rapid decreases in the potassium, magnesium, and phosphorus levels.

 ALERT *Don't hang a TPN solution that is cloudy, has an oily layer, or contains particulate matter. Instead, notify the pharmacy. Also, don't allow a TPN solution to hang for more than 24 hours.*

◆ When discontinuing TPN, reduce the rate by 50% for 2 hours and then discontinue.

Dialysis

◆ Dialysis is used to treat fluid and electrolyte imbalances when other treatments aren't effective in patients with acute or chronic renal failure.

◆ Hemodialysis and peritoneal dialysis are the most common renal replacement therapies used.

◆ Continuous renal replacement therapy (CRRT) is available for some hemodynamically unstable patients.

 ALERT *Because dialysis filters out many drugs, such as antihypertensives and antibiotics, it should be performed before drug administration, not after.*

Hemodialysis

Hemodialysis involves filtering the patient's blood outside the body through a semipermeable membrane that serves as an artificial kidney. This dialytic therapy requires access to the patient's circulation, a mechanism for transporting blood to and from the dialyzer, and a dialyzer that acts as a blood filter.

Advantages

◆ Effectively clears fluid and toxins from blood.

◆ Requires no surgery because temporary vascular access can readily be established.

◆ Offers a short treatment time (usually 4 hours).

Disadvantages

◆ Can cause hemodynamic changes, which means it can't be used for hemodynamically unstable patients.

◆ Produces adverse reactions, such as muscle cramping, and complications of vascular access, such as clotting, infection, and bleeding.

◆ Must be done three times a week.

◆ Demands greater dietary and fluid restrictions than peritoneal dialysis does.

A LOOK AT HEMODIALYSIS

Hemodialysis is a process that filters the patient's blood outside of the body, as shown below. The blood passes through a dialyzer, which removes excess fluid and waste products. Then the blood is returned to the patient's circulation. A dialysate solution is used in this circuit to enhance the removal of waste products.

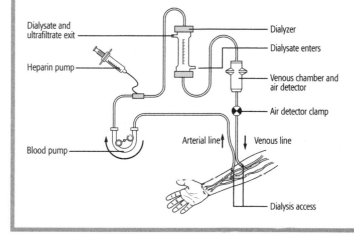

Peritoneal dialysis

This dialytic therapy involves using the peritoneal cavity as a filter. Through osmosis and diffusion, toxins move from the capillaries into dialysate solution (dextrose solution) instilled into the peritoneal cavity. Then the toxin-laden dialysate is removed.

Advantages

◆ Causes few hemodynamic complications.
◆ Allows increased flexibility in the patient's lifestyle and schedule because patients can perform this therapy at home.
◆ Allows more liberal fluid and dietary restrictions than hemodialysis does.

Disadvantages

◆ Can't be performed immediately after surgical placement of the peritoneal dialysis catheter, which requires 2 weeks of healing to prevent leakage.
◆ Causes such complications as protein loss, bowel perforation, peritonitis, and hyperglycemia (from the dextrose solution).
◆ Isn't an option if the patient has extensive peritoneal adhesions from surgery.

UNDERSTANDING PERITONEAL DIALYSIS

In peritoneal dialysis, the peritoneal cavity is used as a filer or natural dialyzer. In this continuous dialytic therapy, a dialysate (dextrose) solution is instilled into the peritoneal cavity through a peritoneal dialysis catheter, which extends from the abdominal wall into the peritoneal cavity, as shown here. At the end of the prescribed dwell time, the dialysate solution containing waste products and fluid is drained from the peritoneal cavity and immediately replaced by fresh dialysate solution.

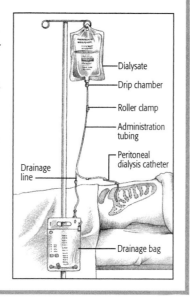

Continuous renal replacement therapy

CRRT is used to manage fluid and electrolyte imbalances in hemodynamically unstable patients who can't tolerate hemodialysis.

Advantages

◆ Allows immediate access to the patient's blood via a dual-lumen venous catheter.
◆ Conserves cellular and protein components of blood.
◆ Doesn't create dramatic changes in the patient's blood pressure, which often occurs with hemodialysis.

Disadvantages

◆ Must be performed by a specially trained critical care or nephrology nurse.
◆ Must take place on a critical care unit.
◆ Requires CRRT equipment and supplies.
◆ May pose issues of staff competency if CRRT is rarely used.
◆ Is time consuming.

FOLLOWING THE CRRT CIRCUIT

In continuous renal replacement therapy (CRRT), a dual-lumen venous catheter provides access to the patient's blood. A pulsatile pump propels the blood through the tubing circuit.

The illustration here shows the standard setup for one type of CRRT called continuous venovenous hemofiltration. The patient's blood enters the hemofilter from a line connected to one lumen of the venous catheter, flows through the hemofilter, and returns to the patient through the second lumen of the catheter.

At the first pump, an anticoagulant may be added to the blood. A second pump moves dialysate through the hemofilter. A third pump adds replacement fluid if needed.

The ultrafiltrate (plasma water and toxins) removed from the blood drains into a collection bag.

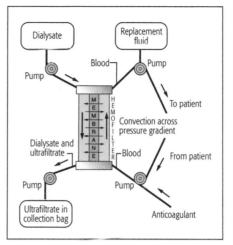

Transfusions

- ◆ Transfusions of blood and blood products can restore blood volume, correct deficiencies in the blood's oxygen-carrying capacity, and provide coagulation components.
- ◆ Depending on the blood product, different blood antigens (ABO blood group, rhesus [Rh] factor, and human leukocyte antigen [HLA] blood group) must be crossmatched to ensure compatibility between the donor's and recipient's blood before transfusion.
- ◆ Transfusion therapy requires knowledge of the types of blood products, appropriate patient care, and techniques for handling transfusion reactions.

Types of blood products

◆ Blood products commonly used for transfusions include whole blood, packed RBCs, granulocytes, fresh frozen plasma, cryoprecipitate, albumin, and platelets.

◆ The patient's own blood also may be stored and administered through a process called autologous transfusion (autotransfusion).

Whole blood

◆ Is rarely used unless more than 25% of total blood volume is lost.

◆ Is available in 500-ml bags.

◆ Treats hemorrhage, trauma, and major burns.

◆ Should be avoided if fluid overload is a concern.

◆ Requires lengthy storage, which may lead to hemolysis and hyperkalemia.

◆ Displays decreased RBC viability and function after 24 hours of storage.

◆ Requires ABO compatibility and Rh matching before administration.

Packed RBCs

◆ Are prepared by removing 90% of plasma around cells and adding an anticoagulant preservative.

◆ Are available in 250-ml bags.

◆ Reduce the risk of febrile, nonhemolytic reactions because about 70% of the leukocytes in packed RBCs have been removed.

◆ Require ABO compatibility and Rh matching.

Granulocytes

◆ Are also called WBCs.

◆ Are rarely used, except in patients with gram-negative sepsis or progressive soft-tissue infection that's unresponsive to antimicrobials.

◆ Require Rh matching, preferably with HLA compatibility tests.

Fresh frozen plasma

- Is prepared by separating plasma from RBCs and freezing it within 6 hours of collection.
- Contains plasma proteins, water, fibrinogen, some clotting factors, electrolytes, glucose, vitamins, minerals, hormones, and antibodies.
- Is used to treat hemorrhage, expand plasma volume, correct undetermined coagulation factor deficiencies, replace specific clotting factors, and correct factor deficiencies caused by liver disease.
- May require Rh matching, but not ABO compatibility testing.
- May cause hypocalcemia when given in large volumes because the transfusion's citric acid binds with and depletes the patient's serum calcium.

Cryoprecipitate

- Is also called factor VIII.
- Is the insoluble portion of plasma recovered from fresh frozen plasma.
- Is used to treat von Willebrand's disease, hypofibrinogenemia, factor VIII deficiency (antihemophilic factor), hemophilia A, and disseminated intravascular coagulation (DIC).
- Requires no ABO compatibility testing.

Albumin

- Is extracted from plasma.
- Contains albumin, globulin, and other proteins.
- Is used to treat acute liver failure, burns, trauma, and hemolytic disease of the newborn.
- Requires no ABO compatibility testing.

Platelets

◆ Are primarily used to treat platelet dysfunction and thrombocy-topenia.

◆ Are also used in patients who have had multiple transfusions of stored blood, acute leukemia, or bone marrow abnormalities.

◆ May require Rh matching.

Patient's blood or blood components

◆ May be banked and used for autotransfusion.

◆ May require the patient to donate blood for a period of time (for elective surgery).

◆ May be withdrawn immediately before the procedure, replaced with I.V. fluid, and then reinfused after the procedure (for non-elective surgery and some elective surgery).

◆ May be used in a procedure that's expected to cause preoperative or intraoperative hemorrhage; shed blood is collected, then reinfused.

Pretransfusion safeguards

◆ Make sure the patient or his next of kin has signed an informed consent form.

◆ Explain the procedure to the patient.

◆ Because the religious beliefs of Jehovah's Witnesses preclude the use of blood products, make sure that refusal of blood reflects the patient's own decision and not coercion by family members or clergy. Consider consulting your facility's legal counsel on behalf of minors and adults incapable of giving their own consent.

◆ Review facility policy for administering blood.

◆ Assess your patient, documenting vital signs and other pertinent information. Notify the physician if the patient has a fever of 100° F (37.8° C) or higher before the transfusion.

 ALERT *Keep in mind your patient's other treatment needs. If he's receiving an I.V. drug that can't be mixed with blood products, for example, plan to insert another I.V. line.*

◆ Check the orders for the type of transfusion to be given.

◆ Triple-check your patient's identity to ensure that the right patient receives the right transfusion at the right time.

◆ Ask the patient if he has ever had a transfusion reaction and, if so, under what conditions the transfusion was given, and how it was resolved.

Care related to transfusions

◆ Maintain sterile technique to protect the patient.

◆ Observe standard precautions to protect yourself. Wear a gown, gloves, and a face shield.

◆ Infuse blood products through at least an 18G or 20G I.V. catheter. Never use a smaller-gauge catheter or needle.

◆ Transfuse blood using a Y-type I.V. administration set (with filter), and infuse the blood over 2 to 4 hours.

◆ After starting the transfusion, remain with the patient and observe him carefully for the first 15 minutes.

◆ Be alert for acute adverse reactions, which typically occur within the first 15 minutes, but be aware that delayed reactions can occur up to 2 weeks later.

◆ Recheck vital signs 15 minutes after hanging the blood, and again every hour.

◆ Use a pressure bag or a specialized infusion pump to administer blood more rapidly if needed.

Flushing lines and using filters

◆ Flush with normal saline solution before and after infusing blood products.

◆ Also flush the I.V. line during the transfusion if the blood is dripping too slowly.

◆ Don't use a dextrose solution, which can cause hemolysis, or lactated Ringer's solution, which contains calcium and can clog the tubing.

◆ Filters work best when completely filled with blood.

◆ Use special filters if needed to trap leukocytes (leukocyte-depleting filters) or tiny clots and debris that can get through standard filters (microaggregate filters).

◆ When transfusing whole blood, reduce the risk of adverse reactions by adding a microfilter to trap platelets.

Getting blood ready

◆ Obtain blood from the laboratory *when you're ready to hang it.*
◆ Check the bag for leaks, discoloration, bubbles, and clots.
◆ Return questionable products to the blood bank.

 ALERT *Don't store blood in a nursing-unit refrigerator because the temperature may be inaccurate, and the blood could be damaged. Blood that isn't refrigerated for 4 hours or more carries a high risk of bacterial contamination.*

◆ Use a blood-warming device and special tubing if the order calls for blood to be warmed before administration, such as when transfusing large quantities of blood. Maintain the temperature between 89.6° and 98.6° F (32° and 37° C).

Giving platelets

◆ Transfuse platelets over 15 minutes.
◆ If the patient's history includes a platelet transfusion reaction, premedicate with an antipyretic or antihistamine, as prescribed.
◆ Avoid giving platelets when the patient is febrile.
◆ Check the platelet count 1 hour after the transfusion ends.

Giving other blood products

◆ Don't mix albumin with other solutions.
◆ Use albumin as a volume expander, if prescribed, until cross-matching for a whole blood transfusion is completed.
◆ Don't use albumin for patients with severe anemia, and give it cautiously to patients with a cardiac or pulmonary disorder because heart failure may occur.
◆ Because cryoprecipitate's half-life is 8 to 10 hours, give repeated transfusions at those intervals to maintain a normal factor VIII level.
◆ Before granulocyte transfusion, premedicate the patient with diphenhydramine (Benadryl) if prescribed, and give an antipyretic for fever.
◆ Agitate the granulocyte container to prevent the cells from settling and unintentional delivery of a bolus infusion.
◆ Give a granulocyte transfusion with an antibiotic to treat infection as prescribed, but don't give it with amphotericin B.

Providing posttransfusion care

◆ Continue to assess the patient as you remove the blood and tubing, and hang an infusion of normal saline solution to keep the vein open.

◆ Watch for signs of circulatory overload, especially in an elderly patient.

◆ Carefully monitor the infusion rate and I.V. site.

◆ Obtain laboratory tests as ordered to determine the effectiveness of the treatment.

◆ For an adult receiving 1 unit of packed RBCs, expect the hemoglobin level to increase by 1 g/dl (SI, 10 g/L) and the hematocrit to increase by 3%.

◆ For each unit of platelets infused, expect to see a rise of 5,000 to 10,000/mm^3 (SI, 5 to 10 × 10^9/L) in the platelet count.

◆ After giving clotting factors, expect to see an improvement in prothrombin time and partial thromboplastin time.

◆ Document blood product administration according to facility policy.

Transfusion reactions

◆ Transfusion reactions may be endogenous or exogenous.

◆ Endogenous reactions are caused by antigen-antibody reactions. These include allergic reactions, bacterial contamination, febrile reactions, hemolytic reactions, and plasma protein incompatibility.

◆ Exogenous reactions are caused by external factors in administered blood. These reactions include bleeding tendencies, circulatory overload, hypocalcemia, hypothermia, and potassium intoxication.

Allergic reaction

This type of reaction is caused by an allergen in donated blood. It may also be caused by donor blood that's hypersensitive to certain drugs.

Signs and symptoms

◆ Nausea.

◆ Vomiting.

◆ Fever.

◆ Anaphylaxis (chills, facial swelling, laryngeal edema, pruritus, urticaria, and wheezing).

Management

◆ Stop the infusion.

◆ Give antihistamines as prescribed.

◆ Monitor vital signs, and continue to assess the patient.

◆ Give epinephrine and corticosteroids, as prescribed.

Bacterial contamination

This reaction is caused by organisms that survive the cold, such as *Pseudomonas* and *Staphylococcus* species.

Signs and symptoms

◆ Diarrhea.
◆ Abdominal cramping.
◆ Vomiting.
◆ Chills.
◆ Fever.
◆ Signs of renal failure.
◆ Shock.

Management

◆ Stop the infusion.
◆ Give antibiotics, corticosteroids, and epinephrine, as prescribed.
◆ Maintain strict blood storage control.
◆ Change the administration set and filter every 4 hours or every 2 units.
◆ Infuse each unit of blood over 2 to 4 hours; stop the infusion if it lasts more than 4 hours.
◆ Maintain sterile technique.

Febrile reaction

A febrile reaction is caused by bacterial lipopolysaccharides. It occurs when antileukocyte recipient antibodies act against donor WBCs.

Signs and symptoms

◆ Increased pulse rate.
◆ Palpitations.
◆ Chest tightness.
◆ Facial flushing.
◆ Headache.
◆ Cough.
◆ Chills.
◆ Fever up to 104° F (40° C).
◆ Flank pain.

Management

◆ Stop the infusion.
◆ Administer antipyretics and antihistamines, as prescribed.
◆ If the patient needs further transfusions, use frozen RBCs and a leukocyte filter, and give acetaminophen as prescribed.

Hemolytic reaction

This type of reaction is caused by ABO or Rh incompatibility. It may result from intradonor incompatibility, improper cross-matching, or improperly stored blood.

Signs and symptoms

- Hypotension.
- Chest pain and dyspnea.
- Facial flushing.
- Chills and fever.
- Burning along the vein receiving blood.
- Bloody oozing at the infusion site.
- Flank pain.
- Hemoglobinuria.
- Oliguria followed by other signs of renal failure.
- Shock.

Management

- Stop the infusion.
- Monitor the patient's vital signs, including pulse oximetry.
- Manage shock with I.V. fluids, oxygen, epinephrine, and vasopressors, as prescribed.
- Obtain a posttransfusion reaction blood sample and urine sample for analysis.
- Observe for signs of hemorrhage from DIC.

Plasma protein incompatibility

This transfusion reaction is caused by immunoglobulin A incompatibility.

Signs and symptoms

◆ Hypotension.
◆ Dyspnea.
◆ Flushing.
◆ Abdominal pain.
◆ Diarrhea.
◆ Chills.
◆ Fever.

Management

◆ Stop the infusion.
◆ Administer oxygen, fluids, epinephrine, and corticosteroids, as prescribed.

Bleeding tendencies

These reactions are caused by a low platelet count in stored blood. The low platelet count causes thrombocytopenia, which leads to bleeding.

Signs and symptoms

◆ Abnormal bleeding and oozing from cuts or breaks in the skin or gums.
◆ Abnormal bruising.
◆ Petechiae.

Management

◆ Give platelets, fresh frozen plasma, or cryoprecipitate, as prescribed.
◆ Monitor the patient's platelet count.

Circulatory overload

Circulatory overload may be caused by infusing whole blood too rapidly.

Signs and symptoms

◆ Hypertension.
◆ Chest pain or tightness.
◆ Increased central venous pressure.
◆ Distended neck veins.
◆ Flushed feeling.
◆ Headache.
◆ Dyspnea.
◆ Back pain.
◆ Chills and fever.
◆ Increased plasma volume.

Management

◆ Slow or stop the infusion.
◆ Monitor the patient's vital signs.
◆ Use packed RBCs instead of whole blood.
◆ Give diuretics as prescribed.

Hypocalcemia

This reaction is caused by citrate toxicity. It occurs when citrate-treated blood is infused too rapidly and binds with calcium, causing a calcium deficiency.

Signs and symptoms

◆ Hypotension.
◆ Arrhythmias.
◆ Muscle cramps.
◆ Nausea.
◆ Vomiting.
◆ Tingling in fingers.
◆ Seizures.

Management

◆ Slow or stop the transfusion if ordered. Expect a more severe reaction in a hypothermic patient or a patient with an elevated potassium level.
◆ Give calcium gluconate I.V. slowly if prescribed.

Hypothermia

This reaction is caused by rapid infusion of large amounts of cold blood. It results in decreased body temperature.

Signs and symptoms

◆ Hypotension.
◆ Arrhythmias, especially bradycardia.
◆ Chills.
◆ Shaking.
◆ Cardiac arrest if core temperature falls below 86° F (30° C).

Management

◆ Stop the transfusion.
◆ Warm the patient.
◆ Obtain an electrocardiogram (ECG) tracing.
◆ Warm the blood if the transfusion is resumed.

Potassium intoxication

Potassium intoxication occurs with administration of stored plasma, which has an abnormally high potassium level. It's caused by hemolysis of RBCs.

Signs and symptoms

- Bradycardia.
- ECG changes such as tall, peaked T waves.
- Muscle twitching.
- Flaccidity.
- Diarrhea.
- Intestinal colic.
- Oliguria.
- Signs of renal failure.
- Cardiac arrest.

Management

- Stop the infusion.
- Obtain an ECG tracing and levels of glucose and serum electrolytes such as potassium.
- Give sodium polystyrene sulfonate (Kayexalate) as prescribed.
- Give glucose 50% and insulin, bicarbonate, or calcium, as prescribed, to force potassium into cells.
- Give mannitol, and maintain vigorous hydration to force diuresis and prevent renal damage.

Selected references

Alexander, M., and Corrigan, A.M. *Core Curriculum for Infusion Nursing,* 3rd ed. Philadelphia: Lippincott Williams & Wilkins, 2003.

Becker, K.L., et al. *Principles and Practice of Endocrinology and Metabolism,* 3rd ed. Philadelphia: Lippincott Williams & Wilkins, 2003.

Braunwald, E., et al. *Harrison's Principles of Internal Medicine,* 15th ed. New York: McGraw-Hill Book Co., 2001.

Cartotto, R., et al. "A Prospective Study on the Implications of a Base Deficit During Fluid Resuscitation," *Journal of Burn Care and Rehabilitation* 24(2):75-84, March-April 2003.

Critical Care Challenges: Disorders, Treatments, and Procedures. Philadelphia: Lippincott Williams & Wilkins, 2003.

Critical Care Nursing Made Incredibly Easy. Philadelphia: Lippincott Williams & Wilkins, 2003.

Fluid and Electrolytes Made Incredibly Easy, 2nd ed. Springhouse, Pa: Springhouse Corp., 2002.

Gould, B.E. *Pathophysiology for Health Care Professionals,* 2nd ed. Philadelphia: W.B. Saunders, 2002.

Ignatavicius, D.D., and Workman, M.L. *Medical-Surgical Nursing: Critical Thinking for Collaborative Care,* 4th ed. Philadelphia: W.B. Saunders, 2002.

Johnson, R.J., and Feehally, J. *Comprehensive Clinical Nephrology,* 2nd ed. St. Louis: Mosby-Year Book, 2003.

Khanna, A., and Kurtzman, N.A. "Metabolic Alkalosis," *Respiratory Care* 46(4):354-365, April 2001.

Mims, B.C., et al. *Critical Care Skill: A Clinical Handbook,* 2nd ed. Philadelphia: W.B. Saunders, 2004.

Morgera, S., et al. "Renal Replacement Therapy with High-Cutoff Hemofilters: Impact of Convection and Diffusion on Cytokine Clearances and Protein Status." *American Journal of Kidney Disease* 43(3):444-453, March 2004.

Nursing2004 Drug Handbook, 24th ed. Philadelphia: Lippincott Williams & Wilkins, 2004.

Swartz, R., et al. "Improving the Delivery of Continuous Renal Replacement Therapy Using Regional Citrate Anticoagulation," *Clinical Nephrology* 61(2):134-143, February 2004.

Teehan, G.S., et al. "Update on Dialytic Management of Acute Renal Failure," *Journal of Intensive Care Medicine* 18(3):130-138, May-June 2003.

Webb, A.R. "The Appropriate Role of Colloids in Managing Fluid Imbalance: A Critical Review of Recent Meta-Analytic Findings," *Critical Care* 4 Suppl 2:S26-32, October 2000.

Index

i refers to an illustration; t refers to a table.

i refers to an illustration; t refers to a table.

---

i refers to an illustration; t refers to a table.

---

i refers to an illustration; t refers to a table.

i refers to an illustration; t refers to a table.

---

i refers to an illustration; t refers to a table.

---

i refers to an illustration; t refers to a table.

WXYZ

---

i refers to an illustration; t refers to a table.